Raise
WINNING KIDS
without a Fight

Raise
WINNING KIDS
without a Fight

The Power of Personal Choice

William H. Hughes, M.D.

Foreword by John T. Walkup, M.D.

THE JOHNS HOPKINS UNIVERSITY PRESS
BALTIMORE

Note to the Reader: This book embodies one approach to raising children. It was not written about your child. While the author believes in and practices its philosophy, he adjusts his approach to suit each child's particular need and each family's situation. Obviously, he would not advise you about your child or treat your child without first learning a great deal about him or her, and so your approach to child rearing should not be based solely on what is written here.

Printed in the United States of America on acid-free paper
9 8 7 6 5 4 3 2 1

The Johns Hopkins University Press
2715 North Charles Street
Baltimore, Maryland 21218-4363
www.press.jhu.edu

Library of Congress Cataloging-in-Publication Data
Hughes, William H.
Raise winning kids without a fight : the power of personal choice /
William H. Hughes ; foreword by John T. Walkup.
    p.   cm.
Includes bibliographical references and index.
ISBN-13: 978-0-8018-9339-1 (hardcover : alk. paper)
ISBN-10: 0-8018-9339-9 (hardcover : alk. paper)
ISBN-13: 978-0-8018-9340-7 (pbk. : alk. paper)
ISBN-10: 0-8018-9340-2 (pbk. : alk. paper)
1. Behavior disorders in children—Treatment. 2. Rewards and
punishments in education. I. Title.
RJ506.B44H84 2009
618.92´89—dc22   2008050490

A catalog record for this book is available from the British Library.

Special discounts are available for bulk purchases of this book. For more information, please contact Special Sales at 410-516-6936 or specialsales@press.jhu.edu.

The Johns Hopkins University Press uses environmentally friendly book materials, including recycled text paper that is composed of at least 30 percent post-consumer waste, whenever possible. All of our book papers are acid-free, and our jackets and covers are printed on paper with recycled content.

To Joseph and Mary

The will stiffens when another would bend or break it, but relaxes in the presence of gentleness.

—Louis Lavelle

Contents

Foreword

It is a pleasure to write the foreword for *Raise Winning Kids without a Fight: The Power of Personal Choice*, by Dr. William Hughes. While there are many parenting books available, Dr. Hughes's book takes evidenced-based principles of effective parenting and packages them into a straightforward, highly readable, and lighthearted text for parents. As Dr. Hughes acknowledges, we have been teaching our trainees the principles of effective parenting at the Johns Hopkins Division of Child and Adolescent Psychiatry for more than twenty years to help doctors help families deal with the common problems that parents encounter in their day-to-day experience with children. What Dr. Hughes has done in this book is to take those evidence-based principles and weave them into a method that families can apply at home. Well done, Dr. Hughes, for translating for us all these important principles!

At Johns Hopkins we teach two critical aspects of effective parenting. The first is understanding how children develop problem behaviors, and the second is developing parenting strategies that prevent or correct these problem behaviors. There are two interactive processes that drive the development of problem behaviors: parent-child *power struggles* and the *lack of parental attention* (that is, poor supervision or monitoring). While knowing how children develop behavioral problems is a good place to start, this knowledge doesn't do much to help parents do a better job. So the key to getting parents on track is to teach parenting strategies that effectively reduce the chance that power struggles will occur and that include as part of the plan a systematic way of paying attention. To prevent power struggles, parents must be clear about their expectations for their child and must embed those expectations in a daily routine or plan. While many parents think their child knows what the parent wants of them, if you interview children, you find out how amazingly unclear many kids are about such mundane routines such as getting up and off to school. The daily routine must also have built within it specific points in time when parents evaluate how the child is meeting those expectations (thus showing that parents are paying attention). Of course the daily routine must also include the core concept of Dr. Hughes's book, *rewards* that drive home the point that the parents are pleased with how the child is meeting expectations.

So how do power struggles cause behavior problems in children? Over time, repeated power struggles in the daily routine essentially train the parent and the child to use coercive strategies for short-term problem solving. For example, when a child is successful in getting a parent to back off an expectation (such as going to bed on time) by "not listening," saying "no," arguing, or—worse—tantruming, the child learns quickly that such strategies are effective and will likely use such strategies again when facing a parental expectation or demand. Similarly, when the parent successfully uses demands, threats, punishments, and other coercive tactics to get the child to comply, the parent quickly learns that such methods are effective and will, when faced with a noncompliant child, use those methods again.

While power struggles are almost a natural fact of life, in some families they become the persistent pattern of interacting that tends to escalate in severity. As neither the parent nor the child really likes the feeling of being coerced in an interaction, over time each will use more complicated and sophisticated strategies to counteract the coercive strategy of the other. So, the first time a child may say, "no," but if next time the "no" is not successful, then the "no" may be emphasized with a stomp of the foot. The time after that the behavior may escalate to an argument, tears, or a full temper tantrum. For the parent, a simple demand will be followed by a firmer tone of voice, a threat of punishment, or maybe even striking the child in anger to get the child to comply.

The following is a very bold statement, but the evidence base for it is strong: *The vast majority (probably all!) of oppositional and defiant behaviors are learned by children in the context of power struggles with their parents.* Children learn (some say they are trained) to say, "no," argue, talk back, ignore, whine, pout, and tantrum in the context of power struggles with a parent. Similarly, all of those ineffective and harmful parenting tactics (like arguing, threatening, emotional and physical punishments) are learned by parents when they are intermittently effective in coercing their child to comply. Sadly, as power struggles progress in intensity, the parent has but one choice, and that is to use some definitive coercive strategy to "win" the power struggle or capitulate to the child. Most parents do not go to the most extreme measures to coerce their children to comply, but as a result many parents often feel as if they have "tried everything," and they feel hopeless and helpless about their child's behavior. These are the families that Dr. Hughes and I see in our clinical practice. Clearly, to prevent or redress behavior problems we have to end the pattern of power struggles—but how? More about that in a bit.

How does not paying attention lead to child behavior problems? Parents' problems with not paying attention can start early in a child's life. All young parents struggle initially to understand their infant's needs for love, food, sleep, and comfort. For parents to be successful with early infant behaviors, they have to be able to pay attention, learn who their child is, what their child really needs, develop an appropriate response, and then time their delivery of the response in such a way as to be effective in meeting their child's needs. The inability of parents to identify their child's needs, and to use their response both to meet the child's needs and to facilitate a child's normal developmental trajectories (such as getting a child to sleep through the night), can result in early problems with feeding and sleeping, resulting in a fussy and difficult infant. Not paying attention to toddlers and preschoolers allows them to "get into stuff," usually stuff that is not good for them. Not paying attention can lead to injuries in the home (such as falls or ingestions) or to playing with dangerous objects, such as toys with small pieces, sharp objects, or hot objects. Not paying attention to school-age children can lead to rule breaking (such as taking things that don't belong to them), inappropriate TV or Internet use, falling under the influence of negative peers, and other problems. As children get older, lack of parental attention can lead to life-altering problems, such as early alcohol or drug use, early sexual activity, and delinquent behavior. The heartache for children and parents associated with these problems may be prevented if parents develop skills to pay attention to their child and provide appropriate supervision.

But perhaps more importantly, parents who pay attention effectively really come to learn who their child is, what their child's needs are, and what the next step is in their child's development. Knowing their child well allows the parent to anticipate and prevent problems and to provide the child in a timely way with new challenges and experiences that facilitate the child's appropriate growth and development. Children benefit from being attended to. Children who are well supervised have the experience of being well understood— that feeling we had that our parents "can see through us" or "know what we are thinking before we do" or "always say the right thing to us." We like to teach that paying attention in this way is part of the important developmental task of building a conscience. Parents who pay attention will "know" when a child is experimenting with the boundaries and rules and will intervene. Importantly, children who are attended will internalize that feeling of being supervised and will make choices consistent with the values that their parents live by. Similarly, when parents attend well to their child, they communicate important information to the child about who the child is. Children who incorporate their parents' positive view of them (the "apple of my eye" feeling) will have a very good chance to develop a positive identity. Dr. Hughes and I often see teenagers who are confused about who they are and who seem to lack a moral compass. As we get to know them and their family better, it is not uncommon for us to observe that the parents really don't know their child well and view the child as a bit of a stranger in the home. This is really tough on children. Children don't do well when they feel like their parents are "clueless" about them and their needs. In this way, paying attention is key to helping children develop a conscience and a positive sense of self.

What, then, is the trick to eliminating *power struggles* and *paying attention*? While imparting knowledge is important, parents really need to involve themselves in parenting activities that teach them what it *feels* like to implement their expectations in a routine and to pay attention effectively. You can talk about how to play the piano or tennis, but you have to practice the fundamentals to master each of those tasks. It is the same with parenting. All good parenting programs have parents set up a daily routine that embodies the parent's appropriate developmental expectations and check-in points for the parents to attend to how the child is doing and to provide appropriate rewards. Embodying parental expectation in a daily routine does a couple of things. It decreases discussion of routine daily activities (decreases chances of a power struggle), so that parents are less "nudgey" (which kids hate), and it teaches children mastery of their own activities and tasks (which kids love). Essentially, when kids clearly know what they are supposed to do, they do it; and when they are doing what they are supposed to be doing, they are less likely to be doing things they are not supposed to be doing. All good daily routines also have check-in points followed by pleasant and rewarding experiences. Check-in points are the designated times for parents to pay attention and are the point at which parents provide access to pleasurable activities. For example, in the morning routine, a school-age child gets up, uses the bathroom, does their basic grooming and dressing, and cleans their bedroom before heading into the kitchen for breakfast. Those tasks are the routine; the check-in point is the entry into the kitchen; when the parent assesses whether the child has done their morning routine in a timely way (check-in point), the parent acknowledges the job well done and provides a pleasant eating experience (pleasurable or rewarding experience).

Sounds simple doesn't it? When it is done well, it is pretty simple. Just like good musicians and athletes make it look easy and amateurs make it look amateurish, parents who have mastered the parenting fundamentals make it look easy. Setting up a solid daily routine, establishing check-in points, and providing appropriate rewards and pleasurable experiences are the fundamentals of effective parenting. Practicing those fundamentals until they are second nature for the parent and child means fewer power struggles and makes parents more aware of their children and how to care for them. (By the way, children tend to get on board faster with the routine than parents.) While it sounds simple, skillful parenting takes time and thought. It is not something that comes naturally or is simply intuitive; effective parenting is a skill that is learned by practicing the parenting fundamentals until those fundamentals are a way of life.

I hope that Dr. Hughes's book will be the beginning of a lifelong journey for parents and children. Parents who read this book and begin to practice these parenting fundamentals have a good chance of reducing current problems and preventing other problems before they occur, but more important, effective parents give their children a chance to have the personal discipline and positive sense of self that is crucial for successful living.

John T. Walkup, M.D.
Professor of Psychiatry and Behavioral Sciences
Johns Hopkins University School of Medicine

Preface

I want to thank the many people who helped me write this book and all of my many teachers over the years. Nearly twenty years ago one of them, a college professor, found out that I was going into psychiatry. He cautioned me then to think for myself and not blindly accept every teaching I might encounter. It was good advice. The common approaches to human nature using psychoanalysis, strict behaviorism, and, more recently, pharmacology and genetics all miss one thing: free will. This ingredient of human nature—free will—takes center stage in this book. In my view, parenting cannot happen any other way.

I have high hopes for this book. I hope that by sharing what I have learned in my work with parents and children I might help the many families I will never meet. I hope that reading this book will help change the hearts of parents and children. There is something here for every parent because I cover situations that come up in all families with children, and I also describe crisis situations that do not apply to everyone. I hope the techniques in this book will ease the difficulties faced by all parents, including foster parents and parents of children with special needs. And I hope that, by showing parents how to work together better, this book will strengthen their relationship with each other.

High hopes indeed. I cast my bread upon the water.

Raise
WINNING KIDS
without a Fight

Introduction

When I present the information in this book to parents in person, they embrace these parenting tools and suggestions with joyful relief. Admittedly, some parents have wondered whether it is a one-size-fits-all approach. It is not. A shoe that fits everyone would be too stretchy to be of much use. But nearly everyone *does* need shoes, since most people have feet. Parents tend to have expectations for how their children will behave. This book points out that parents must monitor their kids' progress in meeting the expectations and that parents must not only provide their kids with the bare necessities of life—they should also reward good behavior and curb the bad. Expectations, monitoring, rewards, and consequences: the ideas presented in this book *do* apply to all kids, whether they have little problems or great big ones.

It comes as a surprise to some people that as a child and adolescent psychiatrist I spend a lot of time working with parents. The way I look at it, parents are with their kids more than I am, and they have a much greater impact than someone who sees their child once a week or less.

In the psychiatric hospital where I work, a sassy little girl—let's call her Kelsey—was admitted for out-of-control behavior. In the hospital she acted fine. Parents always think that a well-behaved act will fool the doctors, but we know that out-of-control kids can adjust their behavior when they want to. I told Kelsey I was going to meet with her grandparents, who are raising her, and teach them how to manage her. She acted shocked: "That's like saying they're really bad parents!" I joked, "It's *like* saying that but it's *not* saying that." I pointed out that golfers take lessons but that doesn't mean they are really bad golfers.

Medicine is art *and* science. The science behind this book is based largely on the research of Gerald Patterson. I learned the principles from John Walkup, M.D., during my training at the Johns Hopkins Hospital. I have been teaching them and using them ever since. The *Journal of the American Academy of Child and Adolescent Psychiatry* calls these evidenced-based principles among the most substantiated in the field. Yet I have seen them work for some people and not for others, and I have wondered why.

Medicine is more than just science. It is also an art. Science cannot answer questions like "Do we have free will?" or tell us why it is wrong to use another person as an object. Science that would treat another person as an object has become depersonalized.

Parenting is also an art. Good art cannot be rushed. There is a voice inside many parents' heads that says, "If you are a good parent, you can get your child to do such and such." That voice creates pressure that makes parents feel hurried. You can't raise kids in a hurry. Obedience, like all good habits, takes time to learn. What I teach parents, and what I emphasize in this book, is the role free will plays in a child's development of good habits. When their freedom is ignored, children find themselves in a science experiment in which they are expected to act a certain way in order to get a certain reward, in the same way a monkey might press a button to earn a banana. I can't tell you how often I have heard parents tell me that rewards don't work. I teach parents how to use rewards *effectively* to improve their children's behavior.

In my practice I also prescribe medicine and have seen for myself how important, even lifesaving, medication can be. But using the principles in this book has allowed me to minimize the doses and number of medications I prescribe and in some cases to eliminate the need for medicine completely.

Getting Children to Behave without Creating Conflict

A doctor's first task is to understand why the patient has come to see him or her. Parents come to me because they are worried about their children. They are worried about their kids' anger and refusal to accept responsibility. Many parents wonder whether their child or teenager is headed for trouble. The book begins by presenting a variety of parents' current concerns and future worries. If the first step in solving a problem is admitting it exists, the next step is understanding the problem in all its complexity. And kids' problems can be complex. Vicious cycles are created when kids take correction the wrong way and respond defensively (and their defensiveness can be passive or aggressive or both!).

Parents end up juggling concerns about their child's self-esteem, having appropriately high expectations, and hoping to avoid conflict. Conflict causes stress for everyone involved. Stress can worsen behavior, and the more kids are corrected, the more they will see it as criticism. Stress can also worsen kids' illnesses. It can impact personality development and may lead to kids' seeking relief in drugs or engaging in other self-destructive behaviors.

The dilemma parents face is how to promote good behavior while avoiding conflict. And that leads us to a discussion of using rewards to change kids' behavior. The concrete result of the techniques in this book is the creation of a schedule of expectations for a child or teenager. Are expectations being met? It is up to parents to find out. Rewards such as a sleepover or a favorite TV show are given only if expectations are met. In this book we will focus on clarifying expectations, when and how to monitor behavior, and effective use of rewards. In this way parents teach by altering the child's environment rather than by verbally instructing—by saying things that the child may interpret as criticism.

We will see how to use rewards effectively *and why up to now rewards have not seemed to work in promoting good behavior.* One of the first points that needs to be made is that rewarding kids for working is not bribery. Giving a judge money to decide a case in your favor is bribery. We are teaching children that work has its rewards. A paycheck is not a bribe, and you don't need to worry that your children will grow up thinking they should always receive something in exchange for any little thing they do. Children need to earn concrete rewards, like watching a movie, before they can fully appreciate abstract rewards like "Thank you!" and "Well done!" Attach praise to the reward, and eventually children will learn to value the praise. Praising kids just because they seem to need praising fosters a false sense of self. Praise that is deserved is fitting and builds self-esteem. Attention from parents is a big reward for kids. We must major in giving positive attention for good behavior, not negative attention for bad.

Parents have expectations for their children as a way of teaching them responsibility. They are concerned about their children's future. The first problem they face is that kids resist their parents' efforts to get them to meet expectations. Parents try using rewards to motivate their kids, but kids may respond to a lost reward by saying, "I don't care," leaving parents with the idea that rewards are ineffective. Parents redouble their efforts to motivate kids by insisting that expectations be met. Kids may respond by becoming increasingly passive and resentful or aggressive and defiant.

It becomes evident that good habits are not being formed. Habits should include producing not only a good final result (for example, a clean room) but also a good attitude and punctuality about it.

What, then, will motivate kids to do what they are supposed to do? The answer is: rewards. So, why do rewards seem not to work?

Many parents suppose that it is up to them to make their child do a task. But this supposition contains a fundamental error that is at the root of why rewards do not serve to motivate. If a person is compelled to do a task whether he wants to or not, an element of force has been introduced. A person who is in a condition of forced labor is a slave. The slave will view her food, clothing, shelter, and even periodic diversions (games, candy) as the conditions necessary to keep her in the state of servitude. A reward system in which a person has no choice other than to earn his reward is not really a reward system in the fullest sense. Thus it is that kids will resist a task despite being offered a reward if they feel that they have no choice but to do the task in any case.

Eventually children (and parents) realize that the children *do* have a choice—they do not have to do the task. The truth is—violence notwithstanding—no one can force another person to do any task. (Putting a child in her room or in the car, like putting a person in jail, is a different matter, as will be seen.) The more force that is used to make a child do a task, such as physically holding a child's hand to make him pick up a toy, the less the child is even doing the task, let alone doing it with a good attitude. The more desperate parents become, the more they want to insist that their kids do as they are told. If parents suppose it is up to them to make a child perform a task and they find they cannot make the child perform the task, they will be frustrated; and no matter how parents hide their emotions, the child will know that they are frustrated. This gives the child a sense of control. There is a hidden (and perverse) reward in manipulating other people's emotions. Children can develop a taste for irritating people and begin to seek out negative attention even at the expense of concrete rewards like a video game.

Once parents have concluded that rewards don't work, the child may end up sneaking the video games and so on, but by this point parents have decided that it doesn't matter because (they believe) rewards are ineffective. Parents have the uneasy feeling that they are somehow not being consistent, but they are not sure what to do. Meanwhile the child has succeeded in

1. avoiding coercion,
2. irritating his parent, and
3. getting the concrete reward.

Good habits are formed by repetition but also by free choice. Replace free choice with coercion, and repetition leads away from the good habit and toward resentment. The solution to many a parenting difficulty seems to fly in the face of common sense. If a child is thoroughly unwilling to do a task but is *doing it anyway*, begrudgingly, because she feels coerced, common sense might dictate that the parent continue to insist until the job is done. But this will not help in forming a habit in the child. It will lead to resentment and, eventually, refusal.

A theme of this book is that if a child is truly unwilling to do a task but is doing it anyway because he feels forced, the parent should not waste precious energy prodding. Prodding will not lead to the good habit. The parent should instead be thinking one step ahead, to the *power of rewards*.

Motivation versus Coercion

A theme that runs through the book is that parents need to judge when they are motivating a child, even with sternness, and when they are coercing. A child's attitude will reflect whether she feels coerced or not.

Parents get distracted by important but relatively minor questions like "Who will do the task if not the child?" More to the point, because they do not fully appreciate that habits are formed through the exercise of free will and instead equate their own competence as parents with being able to make their child obey, they end up using coercion. But the goal of parenting should be a child's character formation, not winning a particular battle. And by not insisting that a child do a task against his will, indeed by not even *wanting* the child to do so, parents achieve the following:

- preserve the value of the reward because the child is free to earn it or not earn it
- avoid becoming frustrated when the child refuses, thus not giving the child the power to frustrate
- focus on extending control over the rewards because ultimately rewards *do* matter

Parents need to control rewards for the same reason that a nation's economy depends on banks' being secure. Rewards need not be withheld for more than a day or even a few hours. The method of removing rewards for weeks at a time belongs to the old paradigm of parents being frustrated and in turn hoping to frustrate the child by removing the rewards for an extended period of time. Our goal is not frustration. Our goal is for the child to do a task *willingly*. That is why the approach in this book is different from any system whose goal is *only to get kids to do the things they should*: forcing kids to do a good deed calls their attention to the force while obscuring the goodness of the deed.

By not engaging in coercion, parents will be decreasing stress in the home environment. Less stress will help kids and parents think more clearly. By creating a schedule of expectations, children will see over time that it is their fault if they don't earn a reward. In creating a schedule we will be able to address problems that tend to come up at different times during the day. Some kids move too slowly in the morning. Homework in the afternoon may need fine tuning . . . or a major overhaul! A schedule will also help parents predict *when* children will try to create conflict (for example, after they are told they did not earn a particular reward). When a child becomes frustrated at not getting a reward, it is evidence that rewards do matter. Telling a child "No" can be a minor crisis. Kids will try to make parents own the problem, but if parents keep their head, they can help guide the child through the crisis.

Parents must not allow themselves to be bullied. Some kids get really angry. We will be talking about how to manage that anger, how to use time out effectively, and when to call for help. Most parents will never need to call 911. They can count their blessings. By using the methods in this book, parents will be heading off problems. But all parents need to know what to do when the going gets tough.

When children decide for themselves that they want the reward, they will know how to get it: by doing what they are supposed to do. They will be exercising their free will and will be forming good habits. Over time, a child will learn satisfaction from doing a good job; after all, a clean room can be a thing of beauty. Kids should be praised and will enjoy the positive attention of pleasing others rather than negative attention from irritating them. And they will enjoy rewards (more than when they sneak them) because they have earned the rewards fair and square. This sequence will build a child's sense of self as being free, being a valued part of a community, and being capable of achieving goals.

We will accomplish all the above while *decreasing* the amount of time spent correcting the child. *A word of warning*: By correcting your children less frequently, you will add weight to every word you do speak. You will have to be more careful than ever that those words build up, not tear down. Kids know how to get negative attention. Once they start behaving better, you would do well to give them at least as much positive attention for the good behavior as they used to get negative attention for the bad.

A Guide to This Guide

Chapter 1 of this book describes behavior problems that many parents will be able to identify with. Chapter 2 spells out just why parents are concerned: their kids' futures are at stake. Chapter 3 outlines some basic requirements in a reward system. Chapter 4 brings us to rock bottom. Nothing seems to work—not rewards, not fighting—and parents feel like giving up but know they can't. Chapter 5 shines a ray of hope as it proclaims that rewards will work to motivate kids if three pitfalls are avoided. Chapters 6 through 10 help apply the theory to real life as they offer guidance to parents on how to create and implement a plan for behavioral change. Chapter 11 addresses problems that come up as some kids resist change. These kids will try to make you feel as if you are making things worse. You're not. Chapter 12 outlines how I present the idea of a behavior plan to the kids I see in my practice as a child and adolescent psychiatrist. Chapter 13 offers reflections on the virtues we hope to instill in our children. The concluding chapter sums up expectations, inspections, lines in the sand, and other concepts covered in the book. (Additional information can be found at www .raisewinningkids.com.)

In this book I refer to "you" as the parent and to "us" as parents. I, too, am a parent. I had the uncomfortable task of calling my daughter's soccer coach and telling him she couldn't participate in a game because of her behavior. I saw the coach months later at a Christmas party. He told me it made his day to know he wasn't the only one with a willful kid. I refer to "kids" and "children" in this book, but the principles apply as much to a five-year-old as to a fifteen-year-old. They apply regardless of whether a child is gifted and talented or has mental retardation or bipolar disorder. The principles apply to any child of whom you have any expectations for growth and development. The examples I use will clearly apply only to some children, but they should help all parents to understand how these techniques work. Parents will need to get their own creative juices flowing to come up with ideas to suit their own needs. The examples I use in this book are from real families, and some of the creative solutions came directly from the parents . . . and some of them even come from the kids.

But first, we may ask whether your child even needs to change. Is your child developing good habits? If every week, every month, every year your child exhibits better, more responsible behavior and complains less about it, your child is developing good habits. If grades are decreasing or bad attitude is increasing, you may have trouble with a capital T. Many children fall somewhere in between. The techniques that I am about to describe are effective for all.

1

When Is a Problem a Problem?

Of course the secret of parenting is love. The question is how to translate love into parenting.

When Misbehavior Becomes Problem Behavior

All kids misbehave, and most of the time it's nothing to worry about. But sometimes it signifies future trouble. Parents wish a happy future for their kids, and so a question on the minds of many parents is "Does my child really have a problem?"

Let's face it, kids can be annoying. They get cranky. They act without thinking. They can be selfish, and they can fuss when they don't get what they want. They have a lot to learn.

Where, then, do we draw the line between normal misbehavior and true problem behavior? The question of how to define normal behavior takes on new life during puberty, when parents wonder how much blame to put on hormones. It is not often helpful to get advice from friends or family, who usually try to be reassuring by saying that their own kids behave the same way.

I draw the line where either anger or avoiding responsibility becomes the main concern. Problems in these two areas may signal bigger problems to come. I will tell you how to handle and how to heal these behavior problems in a way that will appeal to both the tough-minded parent and the tender-hearted parent. Parenting is difficult because we love our kids so very much; we would sometimes rather they walk all over us than make them unhappy by sticking to our guns. But the only way to teach them not to let others walk over *them* is to set an example.

Although all children misbehave from time to time, normal misbehavior can, over time, evolve into problem behavior. Consider the following sequence: When children misbehave, they are corrected. We correct them in order to teach, to encourage, and to help. But when children are corrected, they often do not perceive our words as we intended them. Just ask a child or a teenager how it feels to be corrected. The answers will be almost the opposite of what we as parents intend. Instead of feeling that they are being taught, kids tend to feel that they are being criticized. Instead of feeling that they are being encouraged, children are likely to feel that they are being controlled, forced to do things against their will. Some kids feel as if they are being attacked. The more a child has problems with trust, the more he will question our motives. We can tell our children that we correct them only out of love, but sometimes they feel that we don't love them and that they don't love us.

Right or Wrong, Fight or Flight

When children—or adults, for that matter—want to be corrected, *really* want to learn what we have to offer, they give us their complete attention. A person doesn't ask for directions at a service station only to turn away from the clerk and begin looking through the beef jerky! When we want information, we pay attention, and when we are paying attention, we are primarily using the frontal lobes of the brain. The frontal lobes are involved in the so-called executive functions: planning, organization, impulse control, attention span, and cognitive flexibility (thinking on one's feet).

When we perceive that we are being attacked, however, the first part of our brain that comes online is the limbic system. The limbic system is involved in generating emotions. The word *emotion* implies that we are put into motion. In the case of being attacked, the emotions of anger or fear prompt us to fight or flee. If we think we see a snake, our limbic system prompts us to move away, even before our frontal lobes fully register what it is that we see. Sometimes we realize that "the snake" was just a branch that startled us. The limbic system is not always accurate, but what it lacks in accuracy it makes up for in speed. It helps us to react quickly, and in that way it can be lifesaving.

We can see this fight-or-flight response in people when they are corrected if they perceive that they are being attacked or criticized. Sometimes, children will literally fight or flee from a situation. More often than responding with actual physical fighting, however, they will respond with some display of anger. Like the growling of a dog, that anger is a primitive way of saying "Back off!"

Just as the fight response usually results in a show of anger rather than a physical assault, the flight response is less likely to lead someone literally to run away than it is to bring about some other form of dodging the perceived attack. A typically

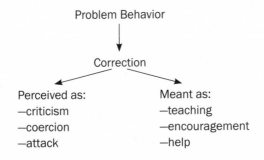

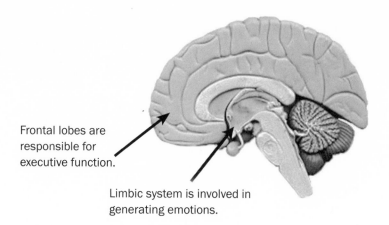

Frontal lobes are
responsible for
executive function.

Limbic system is involved in
generating emotions.

human way to avoid criticism is by denying responsibility. Not taking responsibility is a way of sidestepping and avoiding trouble. Thus it is that at a young age children learn to say "It's not my fault." In their attempts to avoid taking responsibility, children will move from saying "It's not my fault" to saying "I didn't do it." Now we are talking about lying. Not taking responsibility and lying are two points on a continuum of escaping criticism.

We know that criticism can be constructive, but it is very telling that the word *criticism* generally carries a negative connotation. Rather than perceiving criticism as helpful, we have a tendency to see it as an attack. Whenever children are taught something, about drawing for instance, they can see it as an opportunity for learning something new and valuable, or they can perceive it as criticism that something was "wrong" with their drawing. When a change is suggested in how they do things, kids can hear it as help and encouragement to do better, or they can feel they are being ordered to do something against their will or are being told that what they have done is totally worthless. It is precisely when children are hearing the negative message, hearing something bad about themselves, that they respond defensively.

It happens: parents try to be good teachers, and kids get bent out of shape. As long as it isn't happening too frequently, the hurt feelings heal and life goes on.

We need to consider why some kids misbehave more from the get-go.

Temperament, Birth Order, and Stress

If all kids misbehave umpteen (who's counting?) times a day, why do some kids start out life misbehaving umpteen times and then some?

Some kids are born with a difficult temperament. Or a temperament that is just different from their parents'. A shy child with very outgoing parents is going to be pushed. An outgoing child with reserved parents is going to be pulled. Temperament is partly in the genes, and studies show that some people are wired in such a way that they are simply not good at learning from mistakes, no matter how many times they are told.

Birth order can play a role. A young person with older siblings may not start out misbehaving excessively, but that child may develop a bad attitude after being corrected by each parent and then, in turn, by each older sibling.

Life stressors are a double whammy for kids. First, under stress people become more defensive. Stress makes us feel insecure and therefore more sensitive to criticism. Second, stress has a direct effect on behavior. Stress can be negative (as when kids are tired or hungry) or positive (as in waiting for their birthday party to start). Stressed kids are more likely to misbehave and less likely to handle being scolded. In my experience, the most common reason for excessive misbehavior is life stress. Here I include everything that could happen in a child's life, such as the death of a loved one, divorce, illness, and accidents. In addition, anything that causes stress for the parents will reverberate throughout the family. When parents are stressed out, they are more impatient with their children and more likely to frequently and angrily correct them.

Whatever the root cause, some kids do just seem more prone to undesirable behaviors, sometimes from a young age. And the more often a child misbehaves, the more likely she is to be corrected. *But increasing the frequency of correction increases the chances that the parents' words will be interpreted not as teaching, encouragement, and help but as criticism, coercion, and attack.* Imagine an employee in a new job. If his boss gives him advice a couple of times about how he can be more efficient, it is likely that he will feel his boss is being helpful. But imagine the same employee being given advice thirty times a day. That is going to feel like nagging. I witness day in and day out in my practice parents who mean to give good advice and children who feel that they are being nagged. Add "nagging" to the list of synonyms of how kids can misinterpret parents' good intentions. Add "good advice" to the list of those good intentions.

When kids respond defensively to advice or correction, the stage is set for spontaneous combustion. The more kids feel nagged, the more parents will witness their kids' anger and aggression, their failure to take responsibility and lying. But excessive anger and not taking responsibility are *themselves* undesirable behaviors! A problem like being off task gets compounded when a child snaps, "I *was* paying attention!" What good advice can a parent or teacher give to a child who is going to take it the wrong way?

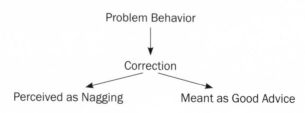

Going in Circles

As noted earlier, I draw the line between normal misbehavior and truly problem behavior when anger or not taking responsibility and lying become parents' *main* concerns. Why do I draw it here? After all, kids can misbehave in such a wide variety of ways, from complaining about what's for dinner to disobeying a direct command. The reason the line is drawn here is that anger and avoiding blame are part of our natural defense system, our system of fight or flight. Trying to eradicate these two problems has a way of causing them to increase. When we correct children for accidentally sneezing on the dinner table, they may respond with anger or by denying that they did it. But now we are in position of needing to correct them for their angry reaction, a secondary misbehavior that increases the frequency of correction! When we pile on the corrections, we decrease the likelihood the child will hear what we have to say.

When a child lies about breaking a window or spilling juice, most parents have the same response. They tell the child that it's better to tell the truth, that telling a lie is far worse than breaking or spilling something. They say, "You'll get in less trouble if you tell the truth." This is indeed good advice. Who could disagree with it? The problem I describe has more to do with the *frequency* of advice than its value. Good advice is meant for the frontal lobes. If people don't want to hear what we have to say, there is little point in talking to them. When we correct children for their angry responses or not taking responsibility or lying, we run the risk that they will respond with more of the same. This aspect of human nature presents a quandary for parents.

Many parents express a belief in the importance of using a pleasant tone of voice with kids. I don't disagree, but I think that suggestion tends to be overdone. It isn't realistic to ex-

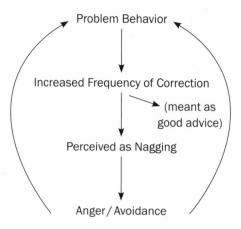

pect yourself to be cheerful all the time. Imagine a coach who has a good relationship with her team. She can scream and holler, and the girls will still like her because they realize that she's encouraging them. However, whether the employer in the example above talks to the new employee in a soft and sweet voice or not, giving advice thirty times a day still amounts to nagging.

When a child responds to receiving advice about lying by telling another lie or responds to being given suggestions on anger management by growing angry, we have that well-known vicious circle. The word *vicious* comes from the word *vice*, a bad habit. Of course, all children become angry from time to time, and nearly all of them will avoid responsibility in order to get out of trouble. The real problem occurs when, through sheer repetition, these defenses become habits. When these defensive patterns become ingrained, kids begin to respond with fight or flight not just when reprimanded but also when they are asked to help out. Just as they perceive correction as criticism, they perceive *direction* not as guidance but as control. They are on guard against ever being controlled. Hence they see even reasonable requests as an attack on their freedom. They even twist the request into criticism, like when you ask a child to pick up a gum wrapper and he responds by insisting that he didn't drop it. (You didn't say he did.)

A stressful event in the past may set off a vicious cycle. I saw a boy who was in the throes of problems with anger, lying, and anxiety. The death of the boy's dog two years earlier was a legitimate stressor, but he and everyone else referred to it as the root of all the problems. Time heals all wounds, however, and by the time I saw the boy, it was his misbehavior and overly frequent parental advice that were causing conflict, stress, and anxiety. My first job was to address the vicious circle, not to pull out my prescription pad.

Another vicious cycle occurs when children develop a reputation either for anger or for always having an excuse. A bad reputation is harmful. Kids with a bad reputation feel they are unaccepted, which leads to depression. A bad reputation puts kids under a microscope: the more closely anyone is watched, the more his or her mistakes will be noticed and perhaps interpreted as more misbehavior. When the gold rock disappears from Room 6, a child with a good reputation will be treated differently than a child with a reputation for causing trouble. Fair or not, a kid with a bad reputation can make people's blood pressure go up just by walking into the room. If parents know their child has developed a bad reputation at school, they may feel they must take a stand against the school staff.

In a certain sense, children can become their own worst enemies: they behave and react in a way that earns them frequent reprimands, yet they are unable to accept or even see clearly their role in creating conflict. And conflict is precisely the outcome. For younger children, that conflict is mostly isolated to the parent who provides most of the discipline. Over time, the conflict involves more family members. Children begin to lose respect, first for their parents and later for other authority figures. Many children I see still behave well in school, but as I point out to their parents, if their misbehavior, anger, and failure to take responsibility continue, their kids will eventually begin to disrespect teachers and other authority figures.

What follows is another link in a vicious cycle: conflict between people causes stress. And stress can worsen behavior. We say that children act out their stress. If they are feeling frustrated, they will do things to frustrate others. It's a pretty sure thing that when children do things to frustrate people, it's partly because they themselves are frustrated.

Acting in Self-Defense and Practicing Bad Behavior

Parents wonder, "Will my child learn to say 'Please' and 'Thank you'?" or "Will my child learn to share?" As long as the child isn't developing a problem with anger and avoidant behaviors, the answer to both questions is yes. But if kids have problems with anger management and accepting responsibility, they will also have trouble learning to say "Please" and "Thank you" for the very reason that they will interpret reminders about practicing good manners as nitpicking, and they won't learn from the correction.

I noted above that the fight defense is hard to miss: the child reacts either with overt physical aggression or with overt displays of anger. Recognizing avoidant behavior can be more difficult for parents. Avoidance can be literally taking flight, as in running away from home or from school. It can be hiding under a desk or holing up in a bedroom. But avoidance may also be pretending to not hear or saying whatever it takes to convince the parent to stop nagging. Small children may burst into tears when they're told not to do something; crying can become a habitual way of avoiding correction.

The fight and flight defenses are natural, but they are also reinforced because they work. In other words, when children behave angrily, most people will give them a bit of space, and in that sense, the anger has done its job. Because it works—in the short term—anger can be reinforced.

The most problematic of the avoidant behaviors is lying. Lying, too, works in the short term. Let us say that Mom or Dad discovers a burn mark on the carpet. When he is asked about it, little Ricky says he doesn't know anything about it. Mom and Dad are stopped in their tracks, and little Ricky's story seems to have worked. All children lie from time to time. When a child is confronted about lying, he is likely to tell another lie. As Sir Walter Scott wrote, "Oh, what a tangled web we weave, when first we practice to deceive." Parents' heads may begin to swim. Little Ricky may seem so convinced of his own story that Mom and Dad wonder if little Ricky is losing his mind or if they are losing theirs.

Parents often tell me that their son or daughter seems to lie for no reason. The reality is that parents just don't recognize the reason. Kids lie to get out of trouble or when they want something. If children lie habitually, it may be that they are caught in a vicious cycle of always feeling criticized. Kids in this cycle get a whiff of danger and quickly come up with a lie to head off the problem. Sometimes children realize *after the fact* that they weren't in trouble to begin with, but by then it's too late. When lying becomes your child's go-to defense, it's a sign that the "practice effect" has come into play: your child has practiced enough to be good at it. Being a good liar means being able to think on your feet. It means being able to head off trouble before it starts. Thinking on one's feet, also called cognitive flexibility, is more a function of the frontal lobes than of the limbic system. When kids become good liars, it means the frontal lobes are working for the limbic defense system. Put another way, their intelligence serves their passions.

The fight defense has an active quality to it, while the flight defense is passive in that it seeks to avoid conflict.

These two defenses can be combined in various ways. That is, people can be predominantly angry even when they are telling a lie. Alternately, people can be passive-aggressive. The silent treatment is a good example. It is primarily passive, but clearly it can be a very hurtful weapon.

The practice effect also comes into play when children respond in anger. On one level the practice comes about because a child with an anger problem is more likely to be corrected for being angry. But the more corrections there are, the more likely it is that the child will respond in anger. Whenever we do anything repeatedly, we develop pathways in the brain. The gate to the brain's limbic system is the part of the brain known as the amygdala, which seems to be involved in our response to fear. Unless the frontal lobes put on the brakes, we are sent into a state of fight or flight. Angry feelings become actions. Like lying, angry outbursts are not something we want kids to practice—nor do we want them to get good at it.

Does the risk of making things worse through frequent corrections or reprimands mean that we should ignore lying and other misbehaving? Not at all, but we do need to provide correction in a way that stops matters from getting worse. We can get kids to behave better by actually doing *less* correcting.

As children's defensiveness becomes habitual, they might feel that they're being picked on when in fact they are not. Rather than living in an atmosphere of trust, these children live in an atmosphere of suspicion, perceiving slights and injustice where none are intended. Children who are suspicious of other people's intentions are apt to say things like "What do you think you are looking at?" Without realizing it, such a child is sending out a hostile message and, like an echo, will likely receive hostile feedback. Because they don't see their part in causing that feedback, these children's belief that people are "mean" is reinforced. Kids like this have a hard time keeping friends because they can dish it out but they can't take it.

We don't come into this world liking to be corrected. At the same time, we want to see ourselves in a positive light. When kids feel that they are being criticized, the defenses come out precisely because they think they are hearing something bad about themselves as persons. As I said before, criticism can be constructive, but the word generally carries a negative connotation. It is worthwhile for parents to make the distinction for kids between an action that is bad and the child who is good. We want to promote that giant developmental step when children are able to differentiate between criticism of *actions* and criticism of *themselves as people*. It is another giant step to be able to welcome criticism as an opportunity for self-improvement.

Building Self-Esteem and Promoting Good Behavior

What is it exactly that the fight and flight defenses are defending? In a word, self-esteem. Parents are usually able to recognize a child's low self-esteem, even though the defiant child or teenager is acting self-assured. Low self-esteem creates another vicious cycle. Girls with low self-esteem may dress provocatively to get the affirmation that they lack. Boys will clown around or take risks in order to fit in. These actions may attract negative attention from their peers and from adults. At the same time, kids with low self-esteem tend to be less open to criticism. They already feel bad about themselves; why would they want more bad news? Parents must be careful in communicating with their children not to accidentally convey the wrong message. One father told me that when he got frustrated trying to help his daughter with her homework, he would say, "It's not like you're stupid." Then he realized she was hearing only his last two words.

The words parents use and how the words are put together do matter.

When a parent tries to help children learn, children often feel attacked, and naturally they resist. When children resist learning, they fall behind in their schoolwork and require more help. The further behind they fall, the less open they are to accepting help. On top of falling behind in their schoolwork and being corrected for *that*, children may be frequently corrected for being angry and acting irresponsibly. As a result, the child's self-esteem is further damaged.

As obnoxious and nasty and unlikable as kids can be when they are angry or sulking or being manipulative, it is important to realize that kids have fragile self-esteem. It is a paradox that the worse people feel about themselves, the angrier they become and the more vehemently they defend themselves, even when they know they are wrong. It takes only a moment's reflection to see that people who act as if they are never wrong are hiding a lack of self-confidence.

Before we look at solutions (and why they haven't worked), we must look more closely at what is at stake if no solutions are found. When we are talking about self-esteem and growing up amid conflict, we are also talking about childhood medical and psychological illness and personality development, which are the focus of Chapter 2.

2

Illness, Stress, and Personality Development

Is it fair to discipline kids for misbehaving when their misbehavior is caused by an illness—a circumstance that is beyond control? Parents wonder how much to blame the child and how much to blame the illness or other stressor, and yet they know they can't give the child a free pass to misbehave.

Children with psychiatric and medical illnesses *are* more apt to develop serious behavior problems. Many kids with learning problems such as attention deficit hyperactivity disorder (ADHD), for example, develop more behavioral problems than can be explained simply by the learning disorder alone. The same is true of kids with a variety of other psychiatric or medical problems: many of them exhibit more aggressive behaviors than can be explained simply by the illness itself. Why does this happen?

It is not uncommon for me to see a child who has been diagnosed with ADHD and whose pediatrician has treated the ADHD with medicine. Many of these children's parents recount a similar story: the medicine helped at first, but then the problems returned, so the pediatrician referred the child to me. One of the first questions I ask is "What are the problems that have returned?" Frequently the most debilitating problem is *not* short attention span, which medication can help, but defiance!

Why do children with learning disabilities and psychiatric or medical illnesses tend to develop an excess of behavior problems over and above what can be explained by the illness alone? What do I mean by an excess of behavior problems? Consider, first, behaviors that would *not* be considered excessive. It would be understandable if a child with ADHD needed to be reminded to stay on task. His being off task is not excessive—it is part of his learning disorder. It would not be considered excessive if a child with a medical illness is short tempered when she is experiencing bad symptoms of her illness. Similarly, a child with an anxiety disorder might be expected to be afraid of leaving her parents. In the context of the anxiety disorder, her behavior is predictable. Still, these behaviors—being off task or irritable or being afraid to leave one's parents—are certainly not desirable behaviors. And there's the rub: anything that increases the likelihood of an undesirable behavior increases the likelihood of correction. The child who is off task will be reminded not to daydream. The grumpy child will be asked to be patient and cheer up. The anxious one will be encouraged.

Parents intend to offer their children teaching, encouragement, and help. But the more often a child exhibits undesirable behavior, the more often the child will be corrected. The more often a child is corrected, the more likely the child will interpret the correction in the wrong way: not as teaching, encouragement, and help but as criticism, coercion, and attack.

Another vicious cycle occurs because stress also affects biology. Headaches, high blood pressure, weight gain, asthma, skin conditions—all are exacerbated by stress. A clear connection exists between stress and depression in children and adolescents. Repetitive stressors also contribute to anxiety disorders. Worsening depression and anxiety do not improve behavior. Stress can cause anyone to feel restless and have difficulty paying attention, thus mimicking or worsening symptoms of ADHD. Therefore, one very important point is the difficulty, even impossibility, of effectively treating illnesses such as ADHD or bipolar disorder or major depression or an anxiety disorder with medication while stress is continuing to make the illness worse. There is also evidence that stress can cause certain genes to express themselves that would not otherwise be expressed. In other words, it is possible that with better stress management certain disorders would not appear at all.

How Do Illness and Stress Shape a Child's Personality?

By affecting kids' self-esteem, these cycles are influencing their personality development. Once patterns of behavior become established, they not only occur in response to criticism but also take on a life of their own. In the case of low self-esteem, misery loves company, and children begin to insult others as a way of handling their own lack of self-esteem. Instead of focusing on their future goals, kids see life through a lens that looks for people who can be manipulated. Kids begin to stir up trouble. They even seem to seek it out. I call this an addiction to conflict, and some kids are junkies. Kids who habitually respond with anger, arguing, and denying responsibility and actively seek to annoy others are going to meet criteria for a diagnosis of oppositional defiant disorder. Oppositional defiant disorder (ODD) is less an illness and more a matter of habit. The treatment for it is behavior modification therapy (discussed later in the book).

Over time, anger and avoidance and lying can change from being defenses to being offenses. In other words, children learn to use anger and deceit not only to defend themselves but also to get what they want. The more kids use aggression and deceit in a premeditated fashion, the more they fit a diagnosis of conduct disorder. Obviously, conduct disorder is not a diagnosis that parents want to hear, but conduct disorder is not lung cancer, and it is treatable. Untreated, however, conduct disorder can develop into antisocial personality disorder, when aggressive impulses become cloaked inside a smooth and deceitful exterior.

For kids who are addicted to conflict, their perceptions of people and things are unduly influenced by fight-or-flight thinking. Life for them is black or white. They overvalue things and people one minute and hate them the next. One minute they think they know everything; the next minute they hate themselves. When these characteristics crystallize, the person is said to have borderline personality disorder.

Kids who get used to a high level of stress are more likely to develop addictive behaviors such as substance abuse and self-injurious behaviors like cutting themselves. Some stress can be good; it can be motivating or exciting. Without any stress at all, people get bored. When people are bored, they look for excitement, which is just positive stress. When we feel too much stress, we look for ways to relax. When kids have grown accustomed to a high stress level, it feels normal to them. Anything less feels boring. A low-stress activity, like playing cards with the family, is intolerably dull for stressed kids.

Yet even though these kids are used to a high stress level, they are also that much closer to getting stressed out. The body can handle only so much stress before becoming overloaded. So these kids are both easily bored and easily stressed out. They are in a precarious situation: They are apt to be desperate for excitement but just as apt to be desperate for relaxation. They already have low frustration tolerance, so they seek out things that are going to give them immediate physiological feedback: food, sex, alcohol, drugs, and cutting themselves. These are things that give the body immediate stimulation. They are addicting precisely because they *work:* they get the job done. If kids are bored, these activities excite them. If the kids are already totally stressed out, these things bring them back down. Kids tell me they cut themselves when they are bored but also when they are stressed out. It is confusing for people to hear that cutting reduces stress, but in a person who is totally stressed out, there is only one way for the level to go: down! Cutting is like cold water. It wakes us up if we are drowsy; it focuses and calms us down if we're agitated.

Kids who cut are often told to find alternative ways of handling stress. A teenage girl was admitted to the hospital for cutting. As soon as I met her, she wanted to tell me all the coping skills she knew as alternatives to cutting, like calling a friend or journaling. But I had to ask her whether she even saw cutting as a problem. She said no, not really.

Before people will stop an addictive behavior, they first have to admit they have a problem. Next, they have to want to stop. A little thing called denial allows people to admit they have a problem but still not want to change. Only after they admit they have a problem and are ready to change will people use new coping skills. But before any other treatment for addiction can succeed, the stress in a person's life has to change. If the stress level remains too high, people will seek relief the best way they know how. The stakes involved in decreasing stress and conflict in kids' lives could not be higher: curing an addiction without decreasing stress requires a miracle. No wonder people turn to a higher power.

Whatever the cause of stress, be it family or school stress on the child, work or relationship stress on the parents, illness, a learning disability, or temperament, a series of vicious cycles begins:

1. A child misbehaves, gets corrected, then responds with anger or avoidance and seems to need more correction.
2. The child takes the correction personally, loses

self-esteem, and becomes even more sensitive and defensive.

3. The child develops a bad reputation and is treated ever more severely or at least is watched more closely.

4. The child's own behavior creates stress that negatively impacts the course of illnesses and personality development.

5. The child begins to seek out conflict but grows ever more desperate in his need to manage his own level of stress.

There is nothing I like more than telling kids I evaluate that I think they are basically normal and that there is help for them. In my experience, the problems causing most of the misery are conflict, stress, and low self-esteem. In this chapter we have looked at what is at stake if things don't change. But in trying to decrease conflict and stress, parents wind up in a dilemma. They want to decrease conflict, but they also want to promote good behavior by having appropriate expectations. Insisting on good behavior can cause conflict, while avoiding all conflict means dropping expectations. In the next chapter we will tackle this dilemma.

3

A Parent's Dilemma
Insist and Cause Conflict or Don't Insist and Walk on Eggshells

Many parents of children I treat in my office and at the psychiatric hospital find that the model described so far in this book puts the pieces of the puzzle together in a way that makes sense—and fits the problem to a T. Taking into account all the elements that go into and perpetuate the vicious cycles described here, where do we start to find the solution? We need a solution that doesn't depend on offering a child good advice because we know that he or she might not listen.

Biological, Psychological, and Behavioral Problems

If a child has an underlying medical or psychiatric illness that can be identified, that illness clearly must be treated. Many parents have discovered that medicine does not entirely solve the problem, however. The system of conflict and stress is extremely complex, so it is hardly surprising that all the problems cannot be solved with medication alone. The problem of vicious cycles is best approached not with medicine or psychotherapy but from a behavioral perspective. This way we can teach by altering the child's environment rather than by offering advice or correction. Our goal is to increase good behavior at the same time that we decrease conflict.

The behavioral perspective looks at behaviors as habits that have developed and can be unlearned or modified using behavioral modification therapy. As we saw in previous chapters, excessive anger and irresponsible, avoidant behaviors are habits that are formed by repetition. A major strength of the behavioral modification therapy is that, while it welcomes input and cooperation from the child, it does not depend upon it. And it's a good thing that it does not. When parents tell me that they have tried behavioral modification therapy but their child refused to participate, I have to smile inwardly. The very problem they are trying to solve is that their child won't cooperate. A chain is only as strong as its weakest link. How can a system work if it depends upon one undependable child or teenager? Remember, we are talking about kids who perceive good advice as criticism and who seem unwilling to learn.

I have seen plenty of kids who have been in and out of psychotherapy and other forms of counseling with the story that they refused to participate. The child or teenager who is unwilling to participate in therapy may be seeing it as more criticism. Kids don't want to be seen as different. Most teenagers don't relish the thought of being in therapy. Kids see therapy as evidence that there is something wrong with them, evidence that they would rather reject. Similarly, children who refuse to take medicine see it as evidence that they are different and "less than." In this sense, the behavioral perspective trumps both medication and psychotherapy because, while it seeks cooperation, it can be employed without out a child's permission.

We are going to develop a plan to promote good behavior. It may seem easier to correct misbehavior after the fact than to come up with a program that promotes good behavior in the first place, but such an approach is short-sighted. Our approach to undoing each of the vicious cycles will first and foremost be proactive. It will focus on promoting good behavior rather than waiting to deal with obnoxious behavior. The more time kids spend being good, the less available time they have to get into trouble. We will indeed talk about handling obnoxious behavior, to the point of considering when to call 911, should that ever become necessary. But we hope to avoid doing that; we hope to prevent emergency assistance from ever being necessary. Therefore, our approach is first of all a positive one.

The series of vicious cycles described above can be thought of as a machine in which undesirable behavior goes in, gets corrected, but due to conflict and stress the result is worse behavior! We want to somehow improve behavior and decrease conflict. Here we run into our first major hurdle, owing to the fact that we have two goals. One is to increase good behavior, and the other is to reduce conflict. If parents' primary goal is to insist on a specific good behavior (for example, cleaning a room), their very insistence can generate conflict. If parents' primary goal is to avoid conflict, then the chores don't get done. In that case expectations are lowered, and parents find themselves walking on eggshells.

Let's take a closer look at this dilemma and how it arises. In real life, there are two kinds of things: things we like to do and things we are expected to do. Work and play, business and pleasure. When I explain this to kids, I just point out that there are things in life that are fun and things in life that are not fun. If you put children in a room with a television and a broom, they are not likely to begin sweeping. Children will choose whatever gives them immediate gratification. This marks a major difference between children and mature adults. To be truly grown up means being able to delay gratification. We are going to help kids grow up not just by giving them good advice but by tending to them like a rose bush. That means raising expectations as the child grows. It means paying attention. And it means using rewards effectively.

Imagine a child who is watching TV. (If your children never watch TV, imagine them wrapped up in their favorite book or another favorite activity.) Mom or Dad says, "It's time to turn off the TV and pick up the living room." Even the child whose frontal lobes are in control of the limbic system is going to feel those emotions to fight or flee. Any child might moan or roll his eyes and say, "Do I have to?" But the children whose frontal lobes come quickly online can multitask. The frontal lobes suppress the emotions to fight or flee at the same time they perform a calculation that takes half a second, a calculation that can be completed even as their emotions cause their eyes to roll or their face to wince. That calculation results in this proposal: "If I clean the room now, can I watch TV later?" A child who operates like that is on the road to success. That child understands give and take and is able to accept the guidance of authority as encouragement to do the right thing now and enjoy the rewards later.

Being asked to do a chore is especially unpalatable when children are engaged in a pleasurable activity. The fight-or-flight children react before their frontal lobes have a chance to come online. They may react with anger by saying "No!" (or with another expletive that means no). They may display avoidance by ignoring you or saying "I'll do it later" or asking "Why can't somebody else do it?" These are the fight-or-flight defenses, and the parent who is faced with them has a dilemma: insisting means conflict, and not insisting means the job doesn't get done.

Parents in this situation are in a lose-lose position. Consciously or unconsciously, the parents are faced with their own choice of fight or flight. Fight with your kids and you generate conflict. Avoid conflict and your kids don't do what they're supposed to do.

In many of the families that I have worked with, years of fighting over chores and homework eventually evolved into parents' giving up high expectations in an effort to avoid conflict. In promoting good behavior, however, our goal will be to raise the bar, not to lower it. We will do this without generating conflict by using the series of steps that follows. The steps may sound like things you have tried before without success. *Many parents have tried reward systems and are convinced they don't work.* There are conditions under which rewards work to motivate and conditions under which rewards actually feed into resistance. The devil is in the details. We are going to see that rewards *do* matter. The steps must be followed in proper order, and any detours must be avoided.

The first step in getting out of the lose-lose situation and actively promoting good behavior is being clear on what you expect your child to do. Kids naturally want to play; we want to teach our children how to work. Parents can and should have high expectations. Having high expectations may create frustration for kids who have low frustration tolerance. Frustration tolerance is like muscle strength, however: the more you exercise, the stronger you become. We develop frustration tolerance precisely by being frustrated and somehow dealing with it. Frustration within bearable limits is good.

Expectations and Rewards

We will spend plenty of time talking about what to do if your child doesn't comply, but don't let that stop you from having appropriately high expectations. You can ask for the moon; just be aware that you may not get it, and certainly not right away.

Here are the essential elements of clear expectations:

1. *Quality.* How good is good enough? The standard you use should relate to the child's age and ability.
2. *Attitude.* A decent attitude is a prerequisite.
3. *Timeliness.* Set a deadline for when the task should be completed.

These elements are meant to establish good habits. They prepare children for future studies, employment, and relationships. We want to teach kids that doing high-quality work is not enough. If a person is a good worker but such a jerk that no one can stand to work with him, he is not going to last long at any job. However, if a person is friendly and outgoing but always late for work, he, too, is going to have trouble keeping a job. Thus, teaching the children in your house about quality, attitude, and timeliness prepares them for life in the real world.

After clarifying expectations, the next step in solving behavior problems is establishing the proper order: expectations must be met before rewards are given. When I meet with parents, sometimes they assume I am talking only about putting business before pleasure, which, of course, they have tried without success. There is more to it. For now, let us simply say that *we know for certain* that trying to push some kids away from something fun (a reward) to something not fun (an expectation) is a lose-lose proposition. In the example I gave of children already watching TV who are asked to pick up the living room or do their homework, I stacked the deck. *Making* a resistant child cooperate is not possible.

We need to begin with a different example—one in which the TV is not yet on and it is clear to both parent and child what needs to be done before the TV goes on. That is, the expectation moves into the Number 1 position, and the reward moves into the Number 3 position. Number 2: the parent checks to see whether the task is done. More on that in a moment. First, a word on rewards and why they don't seem to work.

Rewards and Vigilance

When people hear the word *reward*, they are apt to think of a prize or money or something similar. When parents hear "reward program," they often think of coming up with novel rewards such as giving an extra treat on top of the regular breakfast of cereal or pancakes. This may work for targeting specific problems, such as using the bathroom successfully. But the problem with using novel rewards exclusively is that the novelty wears off. The parent is left having to think up new rewards. Who wants to always be buying prizes? We will discover that the most important rewards are under our noses, and we will find out why those rewards have been ineffective in getting kids to change their behavior. There are conditions under which rewards work and conditions under which rewards do not work.

It is true that rewards should remain proportional to the work. Otherwise children won't find the joy hidden in the work itself, and they will focus on ever bigger rewards. Over time, a child will learn satisfaction from doing a good job.

There is a problem with using rewards that are not already part of the child's daily routine. Tokens, stars or checkmarks, or even money—none of these offer immediate gratification. They are symbols and are meant to be accrued for some long-term reward, something that can *really* be enjoyed. We will want to use long-term rewards, too, but the bulk of the work in behavior change with kids happens in the short term and makes use of rewards that offer immediate reinforcement: things like playing video games and listening to iPods. The rewards that matter most to kids are often subtle and easily go unnoticed. I asked one of my daughters whether she thought her leisure reading was an expectation or a reward. She thought about it and then replied, "Neither, it's just natural." She was not far from the mark.

The rewards that matter most to children are called natural rewards. Rewards are natural if they occur in the normal course of the day. Natural rewards are things like watching TV, listening to music, playing video games, or talking on the telephone. They are things like sugared cereal in the morning, getting money for lunch at school, and getting dessert after dinner. From little things like getting to choose the radio station in the car to bigger things like hanging out with their friends, kids' lives are filled with natural rewards. It is precisely because they are natural and part of the normal routine that these rewards tend to hide in plain sight. The problem with natural rewards is that parents and kids think of them as *natural rights*, and they are not. Furthermore, in the real world of work there are few rewards that come without work. After high school, there is no more free lunch.

If we now have our expectations clarified and located firmly in the Number 1 position, and our rewards clarified and in the Number 3 position, we can talk more about what goes in the Number 2 position. How does a parent know if a kid has done a quality job, with an acceptable attitude, and finished on time? The answer is *not* to ask the kid! Children may think they have done a good enough job. Or they may lie. One of the ways to decrease lying is to stop giving children an opportunity to practice lying. When parents ask a child if a task has been completed—especially when they know the answer is no—they are tempting the kid to lie. Don't ask. The real link between Number 1 (expectations) and Number 3 (rewards) is inspection: checking and seeing for yourself that the task has been completed.

Parental monitoring is required to determine whether a

1. Expectation
2. Inspection
3. Reward

job was done to the parents' expectation for quality, attitude, and timeliness. Gerald Patterson, a scientist who studies child behavior, co-wrote a field-defining paper showing how a lack of parental monitoring is the final common pathway to juvenile delinquency. It is easy for parents to believe children who say they have done their homework, allow them to watch TV, and then get angry at report card time. Not monitoring, then getting angry, then not monitoring, then getting angry again: Patterson calls this pattern harsh and inconsistent discipline. If one of our fundamentals when clarifying expectations is giving a deadline, another is inspection. It should be clear that Mom or Dad will need to do an inspection when the time has expired. Parental monitoring means being there to know whether your child is studying, or checking your child's room to find out whether it is clean. If you discover that everything has been stuffed under the bed when you are kissing your child good night, that's a prime time to think about better monitoring, not a time to shout your child out of bed to finish the task.

Monitoring also means making sure that kids haven't turned on the TV while they are supposed to be working.

Sometimes in my office when parents are explaining the new system to their child, they'll say, "After you've done your job, you come and tell us so we can inspect." Wrong. It's not the child's job to make sure that Mom or Dad does an inspection. Once the new system is established, some kids *will* tell their parents, "I'm done. Come and check." But the burden of inspecting is on the parent. Mom and Dad have to see it as their job.

And will it be Mom or Dad or both of them? The new system works best if Mom and Dad work together. They should be on the same page. If they have vastly different standards or if one rewards the child in secret, they will undermine each other.

One of my patients was a girl who had the task of picking up dog poop, a task she would often not complete. Her mother would let her off the hook, but her father would not. This inconsistency caused conflict among all of them. The girl would pick up only a few pieces, as if that were all she could find. Mom would try to avoid conflict. Dad would get angry. Finally, the parents came up with an agreement. The girl was expected to pick up at least seven pieces of dog poop. Guess how many she would pick up? Exactly six pieces. She knew her parents too well. Her mom, who wanted to avoid conflict, would say, "That's almost seven." Meanwhile, Dad would want to rip out his remaining hair. Six is not seven.

We hope parents are in agreement on what is expected of their children. What if only one parent wants to change a child's behavior? Can a behavior plan still be helpful? Absolutely. Especially if the parent who wants change is the primary caretaker. A behavior plan can also help in situations in which parents share visitation. If kids can learn they can act one way at school and another way at home, they can also learn they can act one way at Dad's but have to behave differently at Mom's.

Before parents can work together on a behavior plan, their marriage has to be in working order. If the wounds between husband and wife are old and deep, the marriage needs some help. When you're choosing a marriage counselor, you can ask whether the counselor believes that marriage is supposed to be permanent, or whether the counselor believes first and foremost that people should try to get all they can out of life. Young couples might be better off talking to an elderly couple who have weathered the storms of married life. If parents are divorced, they need to try to get on the same page as far as their children's behavior is concerned—for everyone's sake.

If children do what they are supposed to do, on time, and with a good attitude, obviously they earn their rewards. But our ship bound for the shores of better behavior is about to run into a squall called "the failed inspection." Before we get there, let's take our bearings. Our first goal is to promote good behavior and avoid the need to deal with extreme misbehavior. Our steps so far have been:

1. Clarify what the child is supposed to do and how long it should take.
2. Determine in advance who will check on compliance.
3. Specify in advance what rewards are at stake.

Before discussing the failed inspection, let us pause for a moment to consider the positive result of a passing inspection. The child has practiced doing a good job; practice makes perfect! He or she gets a sense of accomplishment from a job well done. Parental attention is a big reward for kids. When a child's work passes inspection and Mom or Dad says, "Nice job!" the child is more likely to experience the praise as real, and not as words meant to build up self-esteem. To be effective, praise should be given right away for good behavior: the longer you wait, the less effective it will be. Finally, the child can enjoy the reward in peace, without the uneasy feeling that Mom or Dad is about to pounce because the task wasn't done to their standards. Passing inspection builds self-esteem through a positive cycle of skill building, accomplishment, praise and attention, and harmony: the opposite of the vicious cycle. But what if the job wasn't finished? What if it was done half baked and with a nasty attitude? The failed inspection is the topic of the next chapter.

4

The Failed Inspection

What is the correct parental response to a failed inspection? What should the consequences be? In the real world, consequences are related to the action taken—or not taken. If people are late arriving at the airport, the airplane doesn't wait for them. Pilots don't pretend that they are leaving the runway in order to get people to board the airplane, the way parents pretend they are leaving the park. In college, if students don't turn in a paper or show up for a final exam, they get zeros. The professor doesn't come to the dormitory and try to pull students out of bed. Children need to learn that their choices have consequences.

Some parents ask, "Doesn't yelling work as an unpleasant consequence?" The problem is that it works *sometimes*. And because it works sometimes, the parent's habit of yelling is reinforced. Yelling also gives some kids a dose of excitement: negative attention, but attention nonetheless, which can reinforce the bad behavior. Yelling puts some kids in fight-or-flight mode and reinforces their perception that they are being coerced rather than encouraged. I yell at my kids, but rarely. For yelling to be effective, it needs to be used very sparingly.

So what to do with children who fail inspection?

Using the three steps outlined in Chapter 3, let's assume that you

1. asked your child to pick up his room and suggested that the job would take about half an hour,
2. assured him that you would check his room after half an hour, and
3. told him that he would not watch any TV that evening if his room was not picked up.

If he meant to do a good job but left some socks hanging out of the dresser, that's not a fail. You say "how about the socks?" and your kid fixes it: that is a pass. But what if he *really* failed inspection? Tell him he does not get to watch TV. Then he will either snap, "I don't care!" or just scoff, "Whatever."

If the parent is focused on getting the child to do as he was told, chances are the parent will also snap, "Get back in there and do it!" This sounds reasonable. Parents have the responsibility to raise their kids, and responsibility gives them authority.

If you are dealing with a fairly well-behaved child in a decent mood, one whose frontal lobes are enough in charge that the child can think clearly about the consequences of disobeying, that child may very well "get back in there and do it." Such a child may feel encouraged to finish the task— what she hears the parent saying is, "We both know you can do better, now get going!" Off the child goes. What about our angry or avoidant child? What about the kid who, rather than feeling encouraged, feels forced to do something? In that case, the parent is faced once again with either engaging in conflict so the child will "obey" or avoiding conflict and giving up. This is the same lose-lose situation we faced in an earlier chapter when we asked the children to turn off the TV and pick up the living room.

This is the moment when all seems lost. Fighting doesn't work. Giving up doesn't work. Rewards don't work. Is all hope lost? No indeed, but we needed to reach this place of despair in the book because it is where a lot of parents are with their children's behavior. We needed to crawl in this hole because it is the hole we need to climb out of. What, then, will motivate kids to obey willingly? The answer: rewards. Now we can begin to explore why rewards haven't seemed to work. We will discover three reasons that rewards don't work. Once we cover those reasons, we will see that rewards *can* work, and we will understand the tremendously important role rewards play in teaching kids.

The Proverbial Power Struggle and the Parental Imperative

If a chore isn't done once in a while, it's no big deal. We might even say that if kids do what they're supposed to do 90 percent of the time, they're on track to develop good habits that will serve them well the rest of their lives. Simply stated, habits are formed through repetition. Children who learn the habit of doing good-quality work, and doing it with a good attitude in a timely manner, are on their way to becoming adults who are hardworking and punctual and get along with others. Habits are what make up a person's character, and character is everything. The first reason rewards don't work, however, is related to how habits are formed.

Some kids have problems despite their parents' best efforts, but that doesn't stop parents from wanting the best for their children. Parents can tolerate and forgive a multitude of sins, but they know the world will not be so forgiving. Wanting a child's future to be full of success and happiness is what I call the Parental Imperative. By that I mean simply that no parent who deserves the title thinks, "My child can become a success or a bum. Either way is fine with me." And parents correctly see a connection between the short-term goal of getting a room cleaned up and the long-term goal of becoming a responsible adult. A poster in a clinic where I work quotes Frank Outlaw: "Watch your thoughts, they become words. Watch your words, they become actions. Watch your actions, they become habits. Watch your habits, they become your character. Watch your character, it becomes your destiny."

The Parental Imperative is the long-term goal of raising a child to be a kind and responsible adult by using short-term goals, like cleaning a room. But when that imperative is applied to the short-term goal, a problem develops. Like not keeping the columns straight when doing a multiplication problem, transferring the imperative nature of the long-term goal to a short-term goal (such as doing homework) introduces an error. That error can be summarized by this thought: "If I am doing my job as a parent, then right here and right now I must get my child to clean his room." When parents equate their competence with getting a child to obey, it sets up a power struggle.

Parenting isn't something we want to foul up, and sometimes a voice in a parent's head says, "You ought to make them do as they are told." We adults made mistakes along the way while growing up, and we don't want to mess up our kids. So if that voice says, "You better make them do as they are told," parents figure they should listen to it. The problem is that the voice is wrong. We want to *teach* children to do as they told—and that is a long-term project. *Making* them do something might prove that we are in control, but it doesn't necessarily mean that we are keeping kids on the right track.

As an extreme example of trying to force a child to cooperate, consider the mother who told me about "helping" her daughter pick up her toys by getting down on all fours, putting her hand on top of her daughter's hand and forcing the child's hand to pick the toys off the floor. Ask yourself: Who is picking up the toys in this situation? The bottom line is you can't force a child to cooperate because if it's forced, it isn't cooperation. If you have to use force on your child, your child is not cooperating.

Habits are formed through repetition and also by *free choice*. If a person chooses to do a good deed over and over, he develops a good habit, which we call a virtue. If a person chooses to do something wrong over and over, he develops a bad habit, also known as a vice. But if a person is *forced* to do something over and over, no matter how many times, it will not lead to the development of a habit. Imagine a person held hostage and forced at gunpoint to peel potatoes for two months. That's a lot of potatoes, a lot of repetition. So after being released, forty thousand potatoes later, will that person be in the habit of peeling potatoes? Of course not! More likely, such a person would have a panic attack at the sight of a potato. Even if the person used to enjoy peeling potatoes, that enjoyment would cease when the person became a hostage and was forced to peel potatoes. If the hostage was the best potato peeler in the world, perhaps the only joy in life as a hostage would be to peel potatoes as slowly and clumsily as possible.

Forcing people to do something against their will is coercion. And coercion does not lead to habit formation; it leads to resentment. If the long-term goal of parenting is to help children develop good habits that become part of their character, then coercion must be avoided. *Forcing children to do things against their will does not instill good habits* because children will resent both the task and the taskmaster. A secret of good parenting lies in knowing how habits are formed and recognizing when encouragement is slipping into coercion. Kids don't have to *want* to do a task in order do it willingly. I don't always *want* to get out of bed in the morning but *I* do it; no one makes me. Ironically, once kids recognize that adults are not going to use force, they are actually more likely to comply.

Simply put, good behavior cannot be forced because if it is forced, how can it be called good? What parent is proud and what child is satisfied by a job that is completed through bitterness and conflict? The correct question here is not "Can you force your children to do as they are told?" but rather "Can you *teach* your children to do as they are told?" The goal is a long-term one. Like teaching a child to ride a bicycle, teaching good behavior takes time and cannot be forced in the immediate present. As children get older, parents become more desperate about their kids' behavior. However, fear and desperation will not solve the problem but could make it worse. Saying that a twelve-year-old ought to have good manners is like saying that a twelve-year-old ought to be able to ride a bike. If a child has not been taught how to ride a bike, insisting that the child ought to be able to ride a bike isn't going to make it happen.

Children need repeatedly to fulfill certain expectations in order to form habits, but forcing them to comply leads us away from our goal of teaching them good habits. How, then, can we get them to do things freely? The answer is that kids will do what they are supposed to in exchange for rewards. The key for parents is understanding how to use rewards effectively.

Do It or Else! (or Else What?)

Let's say I want to hire a painter. My expectation is that he will paint my fence. I tell him I will check at the end of the day, and if it passes inspection, I will pay him $400. Now suppose he says, "I can't do it right now. I have another job today." In the real world he wouldn't get the money. But he would still *want* the money, and he would ask whether he could do the job next week. Take notice: so far, the reward still matters! But imagine if I were to insist, "You're not leaving here until you paint my fence. Now, get busy!" At first his eyebrows might go up, but what if I continued to insist? "You're going to paint that fence and you're going to earn that $400, so move it, buster!" I have introduced an element of force. What might he tell me to do with my $400? If he got a call on his cell phone right then telling him the other job was canceled, he still wouldn't paint my darn fence. Sure, he could use the money, but he doesn't want *my* money. Rewards don't work when people feel coerced.

Now imagine things from the perspective of a child: "Mom, Dad, you say the deal is that I clean my room. You're going to check. If I do it, I can watch TV; otherwise, no TV. And that's it? End of story?"

Then the child tests his parents and says, "I won't clean the room."

His parents say, "That's a fail."

The child thinks, "I know it's a fail, and I'm waiting to see what happens."

The parents say, "You won't watch TV."

Child: "I know that part, too. I'm wondering if there's more to the deal."

But suppose that, instead of ending the story here, the parents hear the voice in their heads saying "What are you, some kind of wimpy parents?" So they respond, "Get yourself in there and clean your room!" And the child realizes how the "reward system" operates. The child has discovered the fine print at the bottom of the contract, and it says: "You will do the job no matter what!"

"Get back in there and do it" is the response of parents who think they need to get *immediate* compliance. A parent who begins by saying that the child can pass or fail but ends up *insisting* that the child pass has changed the rules. *The first condition under which rewards do not work is when kids feel coerced.*

Here are a couple of examples:

Morgan is expected to clean her room. Mom and Dad have spelled out what they mean by "clean." Morgan knows that attitude counts, and she is told that she has twenty-five minutes to pick up her room. It is decided that Dad will do the inspection, so after twenty-five minutes, he returns to Morgan's room only to find her sitting cross-legged on the floor in the mess. This is a failed inspection.

Morgan is informed that she has failed her inspection and therefore will not be able to watch TV, play video games, or go to a friend's house that afternoon. She responds by shouting, "I don't care!" This is the crucial moment. This is the moment in which parents are tricked into believing that rewards don't matter. After all, Morgan just said, "I don't care if I can't watch TV or play video games or go to Mattie's house!" But wait! Why did she say that? Does she really not care about any of those rewards? No. She says what she says because she is exercising her free will. She is resisting coercion.

In a power struggle, one gets points for not showing any weakness. But if a power struggle begins, nobody wins.

And power struggles can sometimes escalate into violence, as in the next example. It is important to remember violence is not the answer.

If Mom sees it as an imperative to make Hunter clean his room, then Hunter has a different imperative: not to be coerced, not to be dominated. In this situation, mother and son have opposing goals, as in a soccer match. What started out as a simple agreement—that work should be done before play—has degenerated into a competition. Let us imagine this competition with Hunter calling the play-by-play:

"So, you're saying I can't watch TV? Is that right, Mom? I guess that's one point for you!" If you think Mom really *did* just score a point, you are mistaken. Because next Hunter says, "Well, guess what? I don't care if I can watch TV or not. That's one point for me, so now we're tied . . . and guess what else, Mom: I still didn't clean my room. I'm winning!" This is a competition that no parent can win. For every point Mom scores, Hunter scores two: if Mom threatens to take away the computer, Hunter says, "I don't care and I *still* won't obey."

If Mom gives up and lets Hunter watch TV, then he learns that he can outlast her. If she erupts and beats Hunter into submission, the room might get cleaned, but conflict has won out. Hunter's suspicion that he was being coerced, even attacked, has been confirmed. He *was* attacked. Everyone is upset. His mother has set this example: if you really want someone to do something, get aggressive. Hit, kick, or throw something. Kids who are hit by their parents learn to hit. Room cleaning has become less, not more, of a habit. The overall lesson Hunter is apt to learn is to sneak out the back door when he hears his mother pulling into the driveway or putting the key in the front lock. Maybe he can find some other boys out there who are also alienated from their parents.

As far as teaching kids to obey is concerned, violence is not the answer. It doesn't help matters that advice from relatives often supports the idea that "good parents" can get their children to do as they're told. This advice usually refers to a "good old-fashioned butt whoopin'." I often give talks to groups of parents. At one talk, a man in the audience became more and more agitated, fidgeting in his seat and shaking his head. Finally, he could contain himself no longer, and he spoke up about how *he* knew how to get kids to obey! From his forceful tone it was clear he was talking about physical discipline. A young mother was also there in the audience, and she shrank from him as though she'd just been hit herself. I could only wonder at the violence she had experienced. Here was evidence that the effects of violence can last a lifetime.

Rewards Don't Work When Children Feel Coerced

Good parenting does lead, in time, to cooperation, but co-operation can never be forced. We must put the Parental Imperative back where it belongs: on the long-term goal of character development. Once parents realize that it is not their job to force a child to obey, the pressure to *make* the child comply is off. The pressure to be aware, and to stay vigilant, remains. *The child who "doesn't care" about rewards is the same one who is going to sneak them in ten minutes when the parent's back is turned.* Kids don't care about rewards? If your child doesn't want something right now, check back in ten minutes. I have worked with parents who have a vague idea about offering kids a choice. A child who doesn't want to pull weeds is given the option of washing windows. That is fine as long as the child is willing to do one or the other. But insisting on one or the other does not take into account free will. It would be like the man with the gun telling the potato-peeling hostage he has the choice to dice onions.

Some parents have a difficult time with the idea of not insisting that their child obey *right now*. One mother put it this way: she had to do her job, and her kid had to do his. That is a master-slave mentality. The truth is she has to do her job only if she wants her paycheck. Perhaps that mother resents her job. We want to raise kids who don't resent work and are willing to work hard, not only to earn money but also because they care about excellence. Too many people go through life brainwashed, half angry, half afraid, and muttering to themselves, "Must peel potatoes, must peel potatoes."

The first reason rewards don't work: rewards don't work when kids feel coerced. In the next chapter we uncover reasons number two and three. Here's a clue: they, too, are closely tied to parents' belief that they have to make their kids obey.

5

Why Rewards Don't Work and Why Rewards Do Matter

Nothing in this book is meant to undermine parents' authority. Parents are responsible for raising their children, and therefore they have the authority to make demands on them. Sometimes parents need to inspire their kids. Parents with a background in sales can sometimes use a "soft sell" to motivate their kids, but sometimes they have to use a "hard sell." There is nothing wrong with raising your voice. As I said, I yell at my kids sometimes. Two secrets of parenting are knowing when you have slipped from encouragement into coercion and being able to judge when your child feels coerced. The biggest clue that your child feels coerced is when he or she becomes defensive and moves into fight-or-flight mode.

As noted in the previous chapter, the first condition under which rewards do not work is when kids feel coerced. The coercive interaction evolves into a battle for control.

There is a big difference between encouraging someone and engaging in a power struggle. Parents who engage in power struggles, even if they have the best of intentions, are teaching their children to battle for control. People need human interaction, and if the only way they know how to get it is through friction, then so be it! This can become a very unhealthy way for people to relate to each other. Conflict has a way of becoming addicting, too: kids become accustomed to a certain level of stress, and when it is not present, they seek it out. As mentioned, these kids are more likely to become totally stressed out and look for relief in drugs, self-injury, or other addictive behaviors.

Children who stir up trouble for apparently no reason may be addicted to conflict. The only thing to do is not give them what they are looking for. This means that when children fail an inspection, they should not be "rewarded" by seeing their mother or father "freak out." When it comes time to do an inspection, parents should think about the story of the ranger at the state park who works in the booth collecting the entrance fee. If you drive up to the booth and suddenly realize that you don't have the five dollars you need, the ranger will not yell at you and will not try to shame you. He will just show you where to turn around. But imagine if the park ranger did get angry. Imagine that every time someone didn't have correct change, his ears turned red and he shook his finger, scolding people for being irresponsible. High school kids would drive up to the booth on weekends just to say to Old Bill the Ranger, "Sorry, dude! Forgot my wallet!" and have a good laugh. As they were driving away, they might even wave a five-dollar bill at him! Like many parents I see, that ranger might come to me and say, "I tell you, Doc, these kids are just not motivated by rewards. At our park, we have fishing, we have softball, we have Frisbee golf. They just don't seem to care." The problem is that the kids were never going to the park in the first place. They were on their way to the neighborhood convenience store until one of them suggested they drive by and get under Old Bill's skin. Which leads us to the second reason rewards don't work.

Rewards Don't Work When Kids Get the Hidden Reward of Manipulating Other People's Emotions

It is very unhealthy for children to become addicted to manipulating other people's emotions. In order to combat that problem and create a system based on rewards that do work, a child must sense that, in a certain way, Mom and Dad don't care whether inspection is passed or not. That doesn't mean that parents must fake their feelings if they are disappointed. Parents can say in all honesty that they are disappointed in the lack of effort and sorry that the child won't be earning TV or having any pie. Parents must demonstrate that despite their disappointment they will honor their child's freedom. And freedom means the freedom to do the wrong thing. Parents' disappointment cannot be so over the top that it becomes a reward in itself. But it won't be over the top once parents realize it is not their job to force their child to "obey." Because forced behavior does not represent obedience, and forced behavior does not lead to good habits—it leads away from them. Parents may overreact when their child does not follow through, and then they may feel guilty (or worn out) and create the condition for the third reason rewards don't work.

Rewards Don't Work When Children Get Rewards They Didn't Earn

It almost always happens. Parents are drained from struggling with a child. There is Molly on the phone or Joshua using the video game. They are not supposed to be doing these things, but their parents figure it doesn't really matter. The parents have tried using rewards, and rewards don't work. Taking privileges away now will just disrupt the house, and who needs any more chaos? Once the exhausted parents decide that rewards don't work, they give up and the child gets the rewards anyway!

To recap, here are the three reasons rewards don't work:

1. Rewards don't work when children feel coerced.
2. Rewards don't work when kids get the hidden reward of manipulating other people's emotions.
3. Rewards don't work when children get rewards they didn't earn.

Rewards Do Matter

If you have any doubt that rewards matter, consider that your children sometimes get angry when they hear that they can't have something or can't go somewhere. Rewards do matter. The parent who has come to believe otherwise has been hoodwinked. It is a clever bank robber who convinces the teller and the security guard that he is totally uninterested in the money so that they both walk away and leave him alone in the vault.

Some parents assure me their kids *never* are allowed to get rewards they haven't earned. In these cases, however, the child is usually getting enough of a bang out of irritating the parent to offset the loss. For rewards to be effective motivators, parents cannot use coercion, cannot give the hidden reward of showing their frustration, and must have absolute control over the real rewards, the natural rewards: sweets, all things electronic, and other little privileges.

Kids may get angry when they are told they can't have something. We will talk later about dealing with their anger. For now, enjoy just for a moment the realization that rewards do matter. If they didn't, kids wouldn't get angry at the word "No."

Now we know the three reasons why rewards don't work and we know that rewards do matter. We are ready to begin creating a schedule to help kids get on the right track. By applying the principles we have learned so far to real-life situations, we will encounter some serious questions. But we will find answers, as well.

6

Laying the Foundation for a Schedule

Kids feel coerced, push their parents' buttons, and sometimes are inappropriately rewarded to boot—these are the three circumstances in which rewards don't work to change behaviors. And all three come about when parents think they have to demand compliance. The critical decision parents have to make is how hard to push. If you are dealing with a reasonably well-behaved child—one who is encourageable (as opposed to incorrigible) but has not given a best effort at cleaning the room—by all means, explain the value of excellence: without effort no one wins a victory. If you aren't feeling poetic, just tell the child, "Get back in there and do it!" But for the passive-aggressive child, there are three reasons *not* to order, "Get back in there and do it!"

The first is that it is a return to a lose-lose situation, no matter who "wins." If the parent wins, conflict and stress are generated. If the child wins, he or she is shirking responsibilities.

The second reason is that "Get back in there and do it!" leads down the pathway of coercion. If children feel coerced, even when they give in they are not moving closer to the good habit but further away from it.

There is a third reason for not telling some kids to "Get back in there and do it!" One of the three steps in promoting good behavior (discussed in Chapter 3) is establishing clear expectations about what the child is supposed to do and setting a deadline by which the child was supposed to have it done. Deadlines motivate us. They are the reason kids turn in papers and projects. They are the reason adults pay income taxes on time.

If a child has been given half an hour to clean the room, the parent is obligated to check thirty minutes later. If the job is not done and the parent insists that the child go back and do it, what does that teach the child about the meaning of a deadline (or the meaning of thirty minutes, for that matter)? The child learns that there was no real deadline, no ultimatum. Telling a child to "Get back in there and do it!" after the deadline has expired does not teach a child about time management. It teaches the child he has another opportunity to practice arguing. Nobody needs that kind of practice. Too many second chances teach kids they can disobey, fail inspection, irritate people, do tasks when *they* feel like doing them, and still get all the rewards. Giving second chances is a trap for parents who think the main goal is getting the child to comply ASAP.

You Fail Inspection, You Lose Rewards— but for How Long?

We are trying to promote good behavior in the child who won't do as he or she was asked. Our plan in this situation is to withhold certain rewards, but for how long? The answer is: not for very long. Taking away rewards for too long works against the reward system.

A typical day can be divided into three parts: morning, afternoon, and evening. Children who don't do what they are supposed to do in the afternoon should lose rewards for that afternoon. However, in the evening they should have another opportunity to master an obligation, such as cleaning up after dinner or taking a bath without making a mess in the bathroom. In this way, even if they failed the afternoon inspection, they have an opportunity to pass inspection in the evening.

Children live in the here and now—or at most in the short term. Telling kids that they are grounded from television for days or weeks is problematic for a couple of reasons. First and foremost, it is hard to monitor something like TV watching for an extended period of time, so kids are likely to sneak opportunities to watch. If they are able to watch TV despite the ban, they have no reason to comply with your wishes.

Another problem is that if grounding lasts too long, parents may either forget the punishment or, after they are no longer angry, decide that the punishment was too harsh.

A third problem with taking away rewards for days or weeks at a time is that this leaves the parent with no motivator: the child has already lost the reward. With no immediate hope of earning something, kids are likely to feel there is no use trying. And if too much time passes, the child forgets why he or she lost the reward and remembers only that the parents are being mean.

When rewards are taken away for too long a time, parents can too easily fall back on giving a child something out of guilt or as a peace offering. After misbehavior has resulted in conflict and bad feelings, parents will want to be the first to forgive and do something nice for their child, hoping that the child will show gratitude through good behavior. It is more pleasant to daydream about buying a gift than to consider whether a child is meeting expectations. Forgiving your child is one thing—but problems arise when parents unwittingly reward bad behavior. In other words, what may have happened without your realizing it is that when your child misbehaved, you lost your temper, felt guilty, and ended up buying her something. From a behavioral learning standpoint, the child has misbehaved and has been rewarded—and therefore is now more, not less, likely to misbehave in the future!

To avoid the pitfalls of withholding rewards for too long a time, we will use a system in which rewards are withheld for only a couple of hours. After that the child is given another opportunity to make the right choice.

My approach may lack toughness because it does not make kids do what they are told to do immediately. But my approach achieves better results. And it is tough, because it demands that parents be in absolute control of rewards.

If a bank robber knows how to get into the vault, he is never going to be interested in doing an honest day's work. Children who truly don't seem to care about rewards being taken away from them in the evening may have had their fill of the things that constitute rewards, having watched TV and played video games all afternoon; or they may know that although Mom said they can't play video games, they will be able to sneak them later in the evening. For this reason, I am absolutely opposed to problematic children having TVs, computers, telephones, and video equipment in their bedroom.

Parents are quick to tell me that their kids don't use these things with much regularity. But kids know that they *can* use them. And when parents tell me their children don't watch that TV in their room when they're not supposed to, I ask the parents how they know this for certain. One mother recently assured me she could hear the television because her room was next door. I did not discuss with her whether she always went to her room when her boys were in theirs so she could listen for the TV, or whether she was certain her children weren't using earphones. As a friend of mine has said, "The burden of parenting is on the parents." Parents need to be a step ahead of their children. Until the children can internalize honesty, parents need to enforce it.

If you think there is no way for you to limit your child's access to rewards because of your work schedule, believe me when I tell you that where there is a will there is a way. Quite simply, it must be done if there is going to be any progress. Save up all the energy that you spend trying to get your kid to comply and focus it on this one problem. Don't be surprised if you find you need help from family, friends, or your community. It's OK to need help. When you're able, you can return the favor by helping someone else.

Whose Job Is It, Anyway?

Who will do the job if the child fails to do it? It depends on the job. What if the job was to make the child's bed? Then it stays unmade. What if the job was wiping up the water from the bathroom floor after a shower? Water causes mildew, and people can slip and fall on water. Yes, I am saying wipe it up yourself. The very thought of doing this after you asked your child to do it may make you angry, but I am telling you that this is a milepost along the route to harmony in the family and good habits for your children's future. Here's a common problem: What if the job was feeding the dog? Somebody has to feed the dog. If it was supposed to be the child's dog, find the dog another home. Building your child's character is more important than owning the dog. If you have become attached to the dog, that's okay, too. Just be clear: Fido no longer belongs to Junior, he belongs to you. You may ask how kids will learn responsibility this way. The answer: by seeing that if they don't take care of something— or someone—they may lose it.

What are kids to do with their "free time" if they didn't pass inspection? That's the kids' problem. For now, you need not worry for their sake about what they are going to do if they fail inspection. You need only know and enforce that they aren't going to do or get any of the things defined as "the rewards." This loss teaches basic justice: you get what you deserve.

Children who are not rewarded are not necessarily sent to the bedroom for time-out; that is necessary only if the child becomes obnoxious. (We will talk in a later chapter about how to do time-out effectively.)

Instead of watching TV or visiting friends, maybe the child will choose to read. (But if the child is heavily into sci-fi or mysteries, these books can be put in a "library" and checked out only when inspection is passed.) Maybe the children will spend their "free time" drawing or knitting, unless these are their favorite activities in the world and are therefore a natural reward. In that case, maybe they will go into the backyard and climb a tree or find out what lives under rocks. In this way, discipline turns into an opportunity for the children to expand their horizons. Kids enjoyed leisure time long before TV and computer games. Learning to use their imagination, learning to be self-reliant—these are good things.

Here's another common parental dilemma: if the children can't watch TV at home, should they be able to go to a friend's house or a relative's home and watch TV there? Children need to earn the reward of having friends over and visiting friends, so, no, they cannot go to a friend's house and watch TV. Grandma and Grandpa need to be on board. If the kids are going to their grandparents' house after a failed inspection, the grandparents need to understand why the kids can't watch TV. Another reason reward systems don't work is that kids are getting the rewards at Grandmother's house!

7

Putting Together a Schedule

So far we have explored the concept of rewards and the concept of expectations, and we have stressed how important it is for parents to check whether their expectations have been met before they award rewards. There is nothing wrong and everything right with parents using persuasive, even sharp, words to motivate as long as the child perceives the words as encouragement to do the right thing. A child's attitude will tell you when he is feeling coerced and when he is thinking "How ya gonna make me?!" Rather than engaging in coercion, parents need to be able to stop and focus their energies on keeping rewards from being "stolen." This chapter illustrates some practical applications of these concepts.

We know that someone who has had a stroke or a head injury may need to undergo physical therapy to retrain his or her muscular and nervous systems. To make progress, the patient must have a schedule of exercises and stick to that schedule. Essentially, we want to do the same thing for a child with a hyperactive limbic system. That is, we want to *retrain the child's central nervous system*. Our schedule will be similar to a schedule of physical therapy for neurological rehab, but our schedule will be for behavioral rehab. Our schedule is a series of expectations, inspections, and then free time with or without rewards.

Do kids always have to be on a schedule? Certainly not. There will be long summer days. There will be times of free play that have not been earned by doing any specific chores. But too much unearned freedom creates a problem, especially for kids with problem behavior. A person with a head injury who does the exercises regularly is going to make faster progress than one who does not. If the idea of a schedule sounds dull, consider thinking of the schedule as a map for a journey.

I offer a challenge to anyone who objects to the idea of a schedule: What element would you delete? The expectations? Perhaps the inspections? Or maybe the part about making rewards contingent on passing inspection? What people fail to realize is that the long summer day with no schedule often ends in conflict when the kids don't want to come in for dinner and are not even hungry because they have been snacking all day. The easier the child, the less the parent needs to keep a strict schedule in mind. For the child in need of rehab, however, time with no schedule isn't doing anyone any favors.

Behavioral problems are usually not caused by a lack of understanding on the child's part. Most children are able to understand and parrot back ideas such as the importance of walking away from a conflict. However, what they lack is emotional intelligence, the ability to control their impulses to fight or flee. Many kids are admitted to the psychiatric unit where I work for these reasons: acts of violence, either toward themselves or toward another person; serious property destruction; and running away from home. These problems are related to fight-or-flight reactions. Taken in this sense, self-injurious behavior is aggression turned against the self. I ask kids how they feel the next day about having cut themselves. Very often, they answer, "It was stupid." I tell them they aren't stupid but that clearly they weren't using their head. It isn't stupidity that causes kids to want to use their hands while playing soccer, it's habit. You can meditate all day long on not using your hands while playing soccer, but that won't take the place of practice. A training schedule provides practice and makes it unnecessary for parents to parcel out all that good advice that children take as criticism.

It isn't as difficult to create a schedule as it might seem. Think of how a typical school day runs for your children, beginning with the time they wake up. Children are already on a schedule of sorts. They get up in the morning. They dress. They eat. Most of them go to school. They come home at a certain time. The school day is all about a schedule. Take a few minutes to write out an average day for your child. Kids don't just get up and go right to school. Put in the details. Think about the things they are *supposed* to be doing and also the things they do that they shouldn't be doing. Parents often tell me their kids do "nothing." Kids never do nothing. They sleep or play. They antagonize. Even sitting on a couch is leisure when it is compared with hard work. Our project is to take a close look at the current schedule to see where parents are unintentionally giving rewards before expectations are met.

We want to reorganize the schedule so that expectations are clarified and rewards are given *only* if expectations are met. Many parents become confused about what they can expect from their child, particularly a child with physical or psychiatric disabilities. But if parents consider their child's current activities, they know what a child is capable of doing. Ask yourself simple questions: "Is she capable of bending over, picking up a piece of paper, and putting it into the garbage can?" "Is he capable of pulling a comforter up on a bed?" "Are they capable of getting out of bed and getting dressed when there is something they want to do?" In my experience, very rarely is a child expected to do too much, though occasionally some parents do expect too much of their children. More commonly, the child resists the parents so often that the parents' expectations are lowered, sometimes to the point where expectations are almost nonexistent. This issue particularly affects single working mothers who are not with their children much of the day and feel some guilt about it. They interpret their child's anger as something they deserve, and they indulge their children. If you have to work, you have to work. Kids have had single parents throughout history and they have done just fine, so don't lower your expectations and don't accept misbehavior as being okay.

When parents tell me their kids misbehave at school but not at home, it often means their expectations are low or they tolerate disrespect as normal. In other words, the child *does* misbehave at home, but the parent doesn't recognize the behavior as misbehavior. Children generally behave worse at home than they do at school, but as the behavior problem grows along with the child, the problem seeps into the school day. The answer is not to first change the child's behavior at school but to change the child's behavior at home. With rare exceptions, kids who are well behaved at home do not have behavior problems at school.

In most cases, coming up with a behavioral rehabilitation schedule is no more complicated than figuring out what a child is already accomplishing—that is, getting up, eating breakfast, getting dressed, going to school, and so on—and then arranging these tasks in a way that minimizes conflict. The new schedule never says "Now it's time to argue." When a child picks a fight that cannot be ignored, that is a different matter (and will be discussed later).

The School Day Schedule

We start with a school day because there are more school days than there are nonschool days. To create the schedule, begin by breaking a school day down into three sections—before school, after school, and evening—and working on each section separately. In each of these sections, we will think in terms of getting things in the right order, the order that promotes good behavior: (1) expectations first, (2) inspection, then (3) reward or no reward. If a child starts the day by eating cereal in front of the TV, parents are in a weak position to motivate the child to get ready. A child who comes home and plays for hours may have little motivation to do homework. To remember the elements of expectations—*good attitude, quality work, and timeliness*—think ABC: attitude, best effort, and clock. Parents don't need to do one inspection after each task. Rather, group as many expectations together as makes sense, one right after the other, so that everything is completed that can logically be completed for that part of the day. The task group should be followed by an inspection and then a reward, rather than having another expectation after the inspection. A child cannot be motivated to pass an inspection if more work follows.

To promote early success with the schedule, focus on the minimum expectation for attitude. We cannot expect perfect attitude from the beginning. If your child is groaning, do not react. Just like adults, children are not in perfect control of their facial expressions (if they are, teach them to play poker). They may grimace or roll their eyes or even mumble. The parent who is too quick to say "I saw that!" needs to know about shaping. *Shaping is the principle that behavioral change happens gradually.*

As parents and children become accustomed to the new system, the bar can gradually be raised as the months go by. An attitude that passes inspection in the early stages may not be a pass nine months later.

It is important to get the day off to a good start. The morning sets the tone for the whole day, yet problems can start first thing with a child who does not want to get out of bed. For many of the families I see, the current morning schedule goes something like this: fight about getting out of bed, fight about getting dressed, maybe fight about breakfast and toothbrushing, then fight about getting out the door.

Remember that making children move from doing something they enjoy (watching TV) to doing something they don't enjoy (picking up the living room) does not work very well. This approach can be avoided much of the time, but one situation in which it cannot be avoided is getting children up out of a comfortable bed and facing the harsh reality of life.

So far we've discussed behavior rehabilitation at home, where TV privileges or visiting friends are rewards that can be withheld if expectations are not met. The rubber meets the road when the consequence of not meeting expectations is being late for school. Parents need to see where their responsibilities end and the child's responsibilities begin. We cannot plead or threaten endlessly for kids to be responsible; at some point we need to thrust those responsibilities upon them. The child who swims earns praise. The child who sinks will have additional opportunities to do better. But the child who's always buoyed up will never enjoy true independence.

There are two situations we must cover. The first, which is much more common, is when a child resists getting up and getting dressed but eventually does so. Interestingly, these kids usually get to school on time in spite of their resistance. The second situation involves kids who don't seem to care if they get to school or not. We will deal with that situation later. In neither case are we talking about kids who just need a little coaxing to be out the door on time. If it ain't broke, don't fix it. If morning is not a difficult time, you're doing something right.

Preparing for Kids Who Resist Getting Ready for School

If your child is one of those kids who inevitably get off to school but only after resisting all along the way, you are probably tired of fighting every morning. Let's create a schedule of expectations, inspection, and natural rewards or consequences for this child.

Basic expectations before school are usually to get up, get dressed, and perhaps make the bed. (We will want the backpack to be packed the night before.) How will you know if your child has done these things? That's right, by inspecting. The natural rewards vary from house to house, but one that is commonly overlooked is a hot breakfast or sweetened cereal. (Relax. We won't starve your child.)

Let us begin by clarifying expectations. The question to ask yourself is how long *should* it take—not how long *does* it take—to get up, use the bathroom, get dressed, and make the bed? Well, how long would it take if the child were in a hurry to go somewhere fun? When you consider *that* question, you realize most kids don't really need ten minutes just to wake up. We don't want to allow enough time for the child to start goofing around . . . or fall back asleep. Allowing more time than is strictly necessary may unwittingly allow time for arguing. We do not want to allow time for arguing. We don't want to rush the job, either; we want to provide enough time to do a good job.

For most kids, thirty minutes is plenty of time to get up, go to the bathroom, make the bed, get dressed, and put dirty clothes where they belong. Some kids will need more time, some less. A schedule can be modified over time so that it fits reality. It is a learning experience for parents and kids to estimate how long a task will take them and then find out how close to the mark they came.

Parents sometimes try to wake up their children earlier

and earlier so that they have time to "get going." Unfortunately, this rarely solves the problem. Children are quick to figure out that they don't need to get up at the first wake-up call, and they end up getting up at the same time they always did. All this "solution" does is add forty-five minutes of squabbling between parent and child in the morning. When parents say that their child needs a long time to get up in the morning, I ask them how the child would respond on a Saturday morning if she had to be ready to go with the family or with a friend's family to Disneyland. Even if children are truly habitually slow movers in the morning, this habit can be modified over time. Instead of repeatedly reminding children that they're going to be late, we need to specify an inspection time when everything is supposed to be finished.

The basic structure is the same for young children and older adolescents, and it begins with a clear expectation of when wake-up time should be. We start with a school day because there are five of those days in a week. Even if alarm clocks have failed to solve the problem in the past, they are a good place to start. Alarm clocks function as a symbol that the child is becoming independent of the parent. I know kindergartners who wake to an alarm clock. Because alarm clocks don't always go off when they are supposed to, and because children sometimes sleep through the sound, the parent must make sure that the child is awake. And I mean no more nor less than simply making sure the child is awake. Calling the child or gently shaking the child is usually sufficient for the parent to see some sign that she is awake, even if her eyes never open. Any child who repeatedly twists away from the parent's hand and hides beneath the covers can be assumed to be awake, and the parent's job is done. We want the child to learn to see the parent's wake-up call as a courtesy and a privilege, rather than as an attack.

Once when I was at a conference in a hotel, I asked the concierge to arrange for a wake-up call. I woke up before my alarm clock went off, however, turned off the alarm, and got into the shower. As I was getting out of the shower, I heard a knocking at my door. It was the concierge letting me know that the wake-up call had been made and that I had not answered the telephone. It was the hotel's job to make sure that I was awake. If at that point I had grumbled and growled that I did not want to go to the conference and wanted to be left alone, the concierge would not have stayed and reminded me that I needed to get going and earn my continuing education credits.

Girls who want to shower, do their hair, and put on makeup will need to get up earlier. It is generally easier to get showers and baths done the evening before, so think about a change if your child takes too long in the shower in the morning.

If the morning "task group" is done in the specified amount of time—that is, by inspection time—then inspection is passed. The child might get a choice of breakfast. A boy I saw as a patient early in my career thought that "choice of breakfast" meant he could request eggs Benedict. Since then I have qualified for everyone: choice of breakfast means choice from what is available.

Parents need to realize that Frosted Flakes or breakfast burritos are a natural reward, one of the invisible rewards that are part of the normal routine. If children will not do something as basic as get up and get dressed, why should they get Frosted Flakes? I am not saying not to feed the child, but in our house we offer plain toast—no butter, no jelly—if basic expectations aren't met in the morning. One foster mother didn't want to offer only plain toast because her boy had been neglected by his drug-abusing parents. I had to agree with her. In his plan he could always have butter and jelly, but not always pancakes and sausage. Do what you are comfortable with, but remember: sugar is a big hidden reward. Trix, Lucky Charms, bacon and eggs, or breakfast burritos are rewards that have never been recognized as such by the parent. Because these items take time to prepare or cost a little extra, I ask parents what their child is doing to deserve such privileges. What the child has been asked to do is not terribly difficult—basically, to get up and get dressed.

As mentioned before, the natural tendency with a difficult child is to reduce expectations in an effort to reduce conflict. That trend needs to be countered, sometimes by increasing expectations to an appropriate level, such as adding or reintroducing the expectation that a child make the bed. However, if bed making is not something that is important in the family and especially if the parents don't make their own bed, then find a different expectation. No matter how we look at it, there needs to be some form of expectation for the child in the morning.

Letting children deal with the consequences of their own behavior does not cause eating disorders, but power struggles contribute to children's eating disorders. In any event, we are not using breakfast as a reward because children will be offered breakfast whether they pass inspection or not. What we are doing is recognizing that we can withhold the "hot" part and the "sweet" part of breakfast. People who shudder at the idea of using certain foods as rewards need to consider Martha's mother. No matter how much Martha resisted getting up, no matter what a mess she left, no matter what foul language she used, no matter if she hit her mother, Martha got her favorite frozen waffles toasted piping hot and drenched in syrup. By logical extension, whether or not kids eat their dinner, they always get dessert. Not in my world!

Parents who do not want to use food for reinforcement, or for whom sweet or hot breakfast is not a reward option, can find ways around it. Some kids don't even eat breakfast, at least not at home. Kids who pass morning inspection can be given money for lunch instead of having to pack a lunch. You may want your children to earn the privilege of sitting in the front seat or choosing the radio station on the way to school. Passing morning inspection can earn them part of their allowance, as we will discuss later. Perhaps they can earn a short period of watching TV or a video in the morning.

If parents foresee that allowing a child to watch TV or play video games will create problems in the morning routine, they should ensure that the child is *not* allowed to participate in these activities before school. Remember the lose-lose scenario: once a child has parked in front of the TV or picked up the game console or had Captain Crunch before completing tasks, we have fallen into the classic trap of *pleasure before business*. (For the mornings when no immediate reward or consequence is possible because of time constraints, see below, about long-term consequences.)

A reworked morning schedule might look like this:

7:00	Wake to alarm. Mom or Dad makes sure you are awake.
7:00–7:05	Use the bathroom.

Include details that will be relevant to your child. Write on the schedule: "Don't leave pee on the toilet seat" if that is a problem you want solved. Wiping up pee is the kind of thing that parents end up doing for kids to avoid conflict or because "it's just easier." It would be easier to do a lot of things for kids, but that is not what parenting is about. Parenting is about teaching. And when parents have to wipe up pee, they resent doing it and are more likely to snap at the child when he accidentally spills his morning orange juice.

7:05–7:20	Get dressed. Make the bed. Put your dirty clothes where the dirty clothes go.
7:20–7:25	Brush your teeth (if brushing is done before breakfast). Don't leave water on the sink or toothpaste on the mirror.
7:25	Inspection.

Or, if showers are taken in the morning:

6:45	Wake-up time.
6:45–6:50	Use the bathroom.
6:50–7:05	Get dressed, make bed, put dirty clothes in hamper.
7:05–7:25	Shower. Brush your teeth (if brushing is done before breakfast). Leave the bathroom dry. Hang up the towels.
7:25	Inspection.

We do not leave a five-minute block of time for inspection. It ought not to require more than a minute to check that a child is out of bed, the bed is made, the child is dressed, and the bathroom is clean and dry. If everything is finished on time to your satisfaction and if your child's attitude has been acceptable, the child has passed inspection and can now have the breakfast of choice. If not, the result is a "fail" or "nonpass," and your child can eat plain toast . . . no butter or jelly. Hey, bread is the staff of life. If children refuse to eat, they're not going to starve to death. The same for kids who refuse to wear a coat: they won't freeze. It is better for them to experience a natural consequence than to train their limbic system for fighting.

7:25–7:45	Eat breakfast. Put dishes in the sink. Brush teeth (if brushing is done after breakfast).

You can monitor toothbrushing by smelling kids' breath (no wincing allowed) . . . or by watching. If they refuse to do it, consider moving toothbrushing to before breakfast.

If parents feel they absolutely must make kids brush their teeth, even if that means doing it themselves, I won't argue the point, as long as there are multiple other areas in which the child's freedom is acknowledged. Absolute insistence on a *very* limited number of tasks can add weight to their importance and soften the child's perception of being coerced. In general I am opposed to the idea of holding down children and brushing their teeth by force. That method sets up a pattern of conflict that ultimately leads to problems more serious than cavities.

The threat of more frequent trips to the dentist might serve as a motivator. Rather than making a frontal assault on the child's mouth, drop subliminal comments in your kid's hearing like "The other girls (or boys) at school brush *their* teeth and aren't going to care for my child's stinky breath." You have to believe that children will behave before losing all their teeth; otherwise you are resigning yourself to ongoing fighting. If you are considering braces for your child's teeth, I suggest you do some behavioral rehab before the braces go on because if teeth with braces are not properly and regularly brushed, they develop serious cavities. One little girl I saw was refusing to bathe. Rather than fighting, her parents let her get a little smelly, then told her she would need to be seeing the doctor frequently for health reasons. She decided she would rather just bathe. Similarly, rather than fighting about taking medicine, kids should understand the natural consequence of possibly having to go see the doctor to discuss their noncompliance.

7:45   Take your medication. Leave for school.

Some parents may worry that, despite having a schedule in place, their child won't be ready by the time she's supposed to leave for school. Yet most kids somehow manage to be at school on time, and when they do, the parents are usually convinced that their efforts to rush the child worked. But when the morning's events are dissected, one finds that the child had things timed perfectly. The child knows exactly to the last minute how long to delay before getting up. The child knows how much time can be wasted. The child has come to depend upon the parents' growing agitation as a signal that now the time finally *has* arrived to get dressed and get into the car. This situation is not healthy and needs to be corrected.

The solution is to view the consequences for the child's behavior as the child's problem, not the parents'. Before implementing a schedule, the children will have an opportunity to read it or have it read to them so that they know what is expected and what the consequences are. Pulling on children to get them out of bed is a good way to make them pull the covers over their heads. Why do parents go to extremes to get their children out of bed? Parents unconsciously act as if being a good parent means getting their child to school on time. They think it's a reflection of their parenting ability.

The grain of truth is that parents should *provide an opportunity* for their kids to get to school on time. That's all they can do. They can't make them dress in a hurry. Dressing them by force is the wrong direction. Parents who fuss at their kids all morning become like the park ranger who is promoting the very problem he means to solve. Unless kids see it as their responsibility to be at school on time, they are not growing up. They become dependent on Mom or Dad in an unhealthy way called *enmeshment*. Most kids want to be at school on time. Let them be late. Most schools have their own consequences for tardiness and other misbehavior that affects the school directly.

Some parents are afraid to let their child be late because, perhaps unconsciously, they are worried about some "worst-case scenario." It is often useful to go ahead and consider a worst-case scenario. One usually realizes how improbable or even absurd it is. Imagine the worst that might happen to a child who is late for school: your child will eventually flunk, consequently losing self-esteem, and so will continue to flunk, and will finally flunk out completely until at forty years old your child still lives at home.

Sometimes we try to avoid a worst-case possibility that

in reality is so unlikely that insisting on following our routine makes very little sense. Once we stop and think through what is really happening, we realize that the worst case is absolutely the last thing we need to worry about. Realize that the chances of your child flunking are slim. But also realize that if flunking becomes *your* worry, your child will worry about it less. Most schools are more than happy to promote kids these days, whether they have earned promotion or not. Schools have opted to avoid the conflict created if they flunk a child and therefore—no surprise—they have had to decrease expectations.

Now, flunking in and of itself may not be sufficient to change a child's attitude. In the many years I've used this system with families, I know of only one occasion when parents allowed their child to flunk rather than be promoted. What mattered with this boy was that the flunking took place within an entire system where the boy was shown that there was indeed a new structure in place. He was given opportunities to make better choices, but to make a believer out of him, his parents had to allow him to flunk seventh grade. He did indeed become a believer, and after years of conflict at home and turmoil at school, he began to make real progress.

Passing children from grade to grade when they don't deserve it does not help their self-esteem. Taking a real interest in kids, providing clear direction, holding them to a high standard, believing that they can accomplish what you are asking them to accomplish, loving them enough to let them suffer the consequences, never giving up on them, and praising them when they deserve it—these actions will enhance a child's self-image.

I do not mean to suggest that kids just be allowed to sleep the days away until they flunk. The crucial decision parents always have to be conscious of is how hard to push without slipping into coercion. But in the case of going to school, there is plenty of pressure that can be applied (as we will see in the next chapter).

Preparing for Kids to Be Late

In most situations, once children's minds are cleared of the distraction of the power struggle, they will decide that they do in fact want to be at school on time. The morning conflict may have just been unnecessary baggage. In Plan A, once children know their parents means business, they will take over the responsibility of getting ready for school.

You need a Plan B if you know your child will be late for school when the new behavioral schedule has started. That way, instead of feeding into the conflict addiction, you more or less calmly follow the plan, which might be to let the child be late. Your plan might include informing the school about what is going on. The child, too, should be informed: if the child is ready to go when the car or bus leaves, he gets to school on time; otherwise, it's his fault for being late.

For parents who drive their kids and can afford the time, the simplest thing is not to leave until the child is ready. Another idea is to let the child know your car has two departure times. The first time gets the child to school on time. The other one, half an hour later (perhaps after you drop the other kids off), gets the child there late. Oh.well!

For kids who take a bus, if they get on the bus, they make it to school on time. If they miss the bus, you might take them, but you should not be in any hurry. For older children who abuse the privilege of your driving them to school, maybe they can walk or ride their bike or take public transportation.

One can only hope that children will suffer some consequences at school for being late. It is to be hoped that the school will work with you on this issue. But avoid pitting yourself against the school with your child in the middle. We are focusing on home, first and foremost.

In order to jump-start a new system for a child who is determined to defy the parent, the parent may need to sacrifice by arranging to take a few days off from work. If the child is not ready to go on time, maybe you will *not* take him to school. In that case, the child does not go to school that day, and the parent is home with the child. The day at home may be either a work day or, if the child would refuse to do any work, a sick day, but certainly not a vacation day with television and video games. As difficult as it might be to take a few days off from work to stay home with an obstinate child, getting a child on the right track behaviorally is preferable to always being on time—but only after ongoing conflict.

Kids Who Won't Get Up

I work with many parents who have already taken off a lot of time because of their children's behavior, and they are worried about keeping their jobs. Therefore, sometimes steps need to be taken to make sure that the child goes to school, which sometimes calls for extreme measures.

If a child is small enough and has simply refused to get out of bed, one technique is for the parent to put some clothes for the child in the car, and then when it is time to go, *put* the child in the car and give him a choice to either dress on the way to school or go to school in pajamas. For the rare child who wouldn't mind showing up in PJs, have the school prepared to say that children do not go to recess in PJs.

Something almost magical happens when parents see the light and realize that they don't need to argue with their child. A weight is lifted and parents are set free. They begin to think freely and creatively about natural consequences. The ideas presented here have proved useful, but they are just ideas. You may be able to come up with better ones to fit your child and your situation. For that light to go on, some parents need to consider another "worst-case scenario" and then get beyond it.

What if your child is too big and too old to be picked up and put in the car? And what if your child won't go to school on time or maybe at all unless she is forced? Parents are sometimes afraid they will get in legal trouble for not getting their kids to school. They need not worry. The parents who get in legal trouble are the ones who intentionally keep their kids home to work for the family business or take care of younger siblings.

Parents who are doing their best to get their kids to school have nothing to fear. It is the teenager who refuses to go to school who ought to be afraid. Some schools have truancy officers who will come out to the house to make sure that the child gets to school. In some communities, the sheriff's department may provide the same function, particularly if the department has a mental health liaison. I called the police department once just to be sure I was on solid ground. The dispatcher I spoke with was reassuring. She explained that state law says that kids must to go to school; therefore, it is perfectly appropriate for parents to call law enforcement to ensure that their child attends school. If the child can't be managed after getting to school, see below about changing schools.

Instead of being afraid of the school or the law, put them to work for you. They are on your side. The problem is not that law enforcement itches to put parents in jail. More often, the problem is that they don't want to get involved with what they see as family problems.

Speaking of parental fears, some folks are afraid that the neighbors will call Child Protective Services if their kids scream too loudly. Again, CPS doesn't itch to take kids from their parents. If your kids threaten to call CPS, let them call:

during free time, after they pass an inspection. The same with kids of divorced parents who demand to call Dad or Mom every time they are in trouble: they can call when they have earned phone privileges.

You are right in thinking that some of these ideas sound extreme—they are extreme. Certainly if you do not need to take these steps, then don't. But if extreme measures *are* called for and parents are unwilling to implement extreme measures, they may be resigning themselves and their child to an escalating pattern of conflict and mutual distrust.

Parents should recognize that if their child exhibits certain behaviors, desperate measures are called for. Children who are violent or who threaten violence to self or others, or who engage in serious property destruction, are exhibiting behaviors that require desperate measures. (We will talk about what to do about violent children in Chapter 11.)

The Individualized Education Plan

Our hope is that the school can manage your child, which means that schools have their own expectations and rewards or consequences. If your child is not having trouble at school yet, you are lucky. You have caught the problem early. If your child has behavior problems at school, we hope the school will try to handle it rather than automatically send your child home. Maybe, for starters, your child can lose a recess. Then there are detentions. These consequences are meant to make your child never want to misbehave at school again. If they don't work, the next step is usually suspension or getting sent home from school. For this consequence to curb your child's behavior, it will need to work in concert with a behavior modification plan at home. For kids with serious problems, getting sent home is the reward. They don't want to be at school, so they act out and are sent home. They got what they wanted.

When this cycle occurs, it may be time for a change of schools. This may mean having the child assessed for an Individualized Education Plan, also called an IEP. An IEP is meant to make sure that kids receive appropriate education—and other services—regardless of physical *or* emotional impairments. The Individuals with Disabilities Education Act is a federal law mandating that school districts must provide students with disabilities with free and appropriate public education as well as other services such as counseling.

It is not up to the school staff to decide whether a child should be assessed for an IEP. Having your child assessed for an IEP is your right. To refer your child for an assessment, write a letter to the teacher, principal, or special education representative.

The list of disabilities that qualify a child for an IEP includes autism, visual or hearing impairments, mental retardation, orthopedic impairments, and medical disabilities. It includes speech and language impairments, specific learning disabilities, and a category called "other health impaired," which includes attention deficit disorder. The list of disabilities also includes a category called emotional disturbance. This includes depression and anxiety disorders. It can also include oppositional defiant disorder if the disorder is interfering with learning, if it leads to inappropriate reactions on the child's part under normal circumstances at school, or if it renders a child unable to maintain satisfactory relationships with others at school.

We have been discussing how to make sure that a defiant child gets to school. But kids may also be afraid to go to school. If they are being bullied, that needs to be addressed. If they are just afraid to go, or won't go because they are having such a hard time learning, you should request an IEP. Even if a child is assessed and does not meet criteria for an IEP, he or she might still benefit from classroom accommodations through what is called a 504 Plan.

Nevertheless, changing classes or schools without changing how expectations are handled at home is a waste of time. Unless things change at home, changing schools can just be part of a downward spiral.

Just as changing schools is not enough, neither is changing households. When parents are divorced or separated, a misbehaving child may be sent to the other parent's house. Unless that parent is skilled in behavioral rehab, after a honeymoon period in the new household the old habits of defiance and anger and lying and irresponsibility reappear. And the child is sent back to the first parent's. This to-and-fro is a recipe for creating kids with conduct problems who feel that nobody wants them.

In the most extreme cases, if a child, usually a teenager, cannot be made to attend a school, it is time to consider boarding school, a residential school. State-of-the-art residential treatment provides behavior modification much as we have been describing, but in a locked setting. Here again, the effects of three or nine months spent in a residential school might wear off if nothing substantial changes in the home structure.

If your morning routine reflects the ABCs—attitude, best effort, and clock—we expect that before long your child will get off to school without coercion or fighting. We hope that the school can manage your child throughout the school day. So, then, what's next? That's right: homework. One of the biggest challenges many families face at home is how to handle homework, which is the topic of the next chapter.

8

Homework

If a child comes home from school knowing that she has already lost all rewards in the afternoon because of a bad report from the teacher, the child will have little (and possibly no) motivation to do homework. For this reason, even if a child misbehaves during the school day, if the child is on a behavioral rehabilitation program, we want her to come home to a fresh slate. There are exceptions, however—for a big problem at school, there can be partial consequences; for example, the normal reward for completing homework can be reduced from TV and video games to half an hour of TV only. Or the consequences for misbehaving at school can be levied on Saturday and Sunday, as we will discuss.

The After-School Routine

Let's look at a problematic after-school routine.* The child who comes home and relaxes by getting deeply involved in a game, TV show, or phone call has already received a reward and will have little motivation to start homework. Instead, I recommend that problematic children have no more time for relaxation than it takes to use the bathroom, have a snack, and put their backpacks on the kitchen table. A child's

---

* Single working parents and families in which both parents work may need to adjust the homework schedule. See Chapter 9, which includes ideas for these parents.

particular bad habit, such as throwing a coat or sweatshirt on the floor when walking in, can be addressed in the new schedule by specifying that for inspection to be passed, the clothes need to be picked up.

We want to teach children that homework is their responsibility. Certainly, school and homework are extremely important, but not as important as the child's developing character. If we were to agree that homework takes precedence over character development, then by all means, parents should fight with their child until all the homework is done, even if that means that the parent ends up doing half (or more) of the homework. But if we realize that character development is more important, then we are going to raise children who ultimately take responsibility for their own homework. It's all too easy for children, even those who are willing to do homework, to come home and try to remember whether they have any homework while they are flipping channels on the television. They get involved in a TV program and quickly decide that they don't have any homework, only to come to grief at nine o'clock in the evening when they finally remember tomorrow's early morning test.

Make it easy on your kids by getting the order right. The *incorrect* order is coming home, playing for three hours, and then being difficult about starting homework. Instead, parents must expect that children do homework first, soon after arriving home, and play later. When children get home from school, they often think they need a break. I personally think that this idea of giving a child a long break is overrated. The typical school day holds a lot of dead time, and in any event, the child has been out of school for at least a half hour, riding the bus or subway home, walking, or riding in a car. For our purposes, if a child comes home and is able to play for an extended period of time, a situation is created in which the parent is now "behind the eight ball," telling the child to stop playing and start doing homework.

Homework logs, too, can put the parent behind the eight ball. I am all for helping a youngster get organized, but I urge caution where homework logs are concerned. They work this way: parents expect a child to record his assignments in a log and have each teacher initial that he has indeed written down the correct assignment, so Mom and Dad can know what their child is supposed to be working on. But for challenging kids, carrying, using, and monitoring a homework log can provide more details to fight about. And, as noted above, it is the child's, not the parent's, responsibility to know what his or her homework assignments are—and to complete them on time.

Introducing the Concept of Study Time

For children who are particularly headstrong about homework, consider the following method: depending upon the age of the child, come up with a block of time, approximately ten minutes per grade in school, during which the child is expected to do homework. For a first grader, this might be ten or fifteen minutes; for a fourth grader it might be thirty to forty minutes. Ask the teacher or school counselor how much time your child should be expected to study each day.

Rather than calling this "homework time," we want to think of it as "study time." That way, when children say that they don't have any homework, it doesn't change anything. They can use the time to study for a test. If they have no tests, they can work on projects. If they have no projects, they can read. The expectation of putting in the time always remains the same. If a child attends a school that really does not assign any homework, you can still expect a block of studying. Some teachers don't give homework because they know it causes conflict at home. The method we are using allows you to expect your child to study without fighting about it. (By the way, these recommendations are not intended for children who come home every day and responsibly complete their homework.)

Expecting children to study for a specified amount of time means that parents don't have to become private investigators whose job it is to find out what the homework assignments are each day. After all, it's the child's homework, not the parent's. What the parent *can* be responsible for is providing the child with a defined time and a quiet atmosphere with no TV blaring in the other room. Providing time and quiet space for studying shows the child that the family values homework. Any child who has been getting poor grades should see an improvement after coming home and studying five days a week, week after week.

Helping Kids with Their Homework

Some children might need a great deal of guidance at study time. If children need help and can ask for it appropriately, then there is no problem in giving the help. However, if the help turns into the parents once again battling for control with the child, Mom or Dad has become part of the problem. What begins as a helpful explanation by the parent can easily change into a situation in which the parent is demanding that the child pay attention. Parents start out being the tutor but end up being the dictator. It is tempting to insist that the child accept help, but during homework time we want the child's frontal lobes to be working, not his limbic system. If a child asks for help and then becomes angry with the parent, the parent should walk away. Parents are there to help, not to fight. Walking away confirms that the homework is the child's responsibility, not the parent's.

One reason that children's frontal lobes don't get turned on during homework is that they are in the habit of asking for help. They don't look long and hard enough at the work to realize that they *can* figure it out. Giving children a block of time in which they are expected to work serves to counteract this problem. It also counteracts the problem of children rushing through their work. If children know that rushing is not going to get them to the video games any faster, they will focus better.

For children who become particularly argumentative at homework time, try the following: if the total study time is one hour, the child can be expected to work independently for forty-five minutes and may ask for help in the last fifteen. The point here is that if a child believes that she is not able to do a particular problem, she ought to go on to the next one. If she can't do a certain assignment, she can try her hand at a different one. She can even read a book, but she won't get any help until the last fifteen minutes. This waiting period encourages children to focus on their work rather than focusing on the parent. It also encourages appreciation for the help they get; they begin to see it as a real favor or privilege. Imagine getting gratitude from your children for helping with their homework! When parents cannot help with homework because they themselves don't understand it, their children still benefit from the habit of studying, and they can ask the teacher for help the next day.

Implementing Study Time

Parents provide a specific time for study and minimal assistance if the child asks for help and if he accepts help graciously. Parents also need to consider where children do their homework. If children do their homework in their bedroom, parents have no idea what the child actually does during study time. When it comes to homework, parents need to focus not so much on whether the task is completed but on whether the child works diligently. Because the parent is supposed to be monitoring how the child spends study time, the kitchen table may be the most appropriate place for the child to do homework. The expectation for homework time might include repacking the backpack and hanging it up, perhaps on the child's bedroom door, when study time is over. Doing this task at the end of study time eliminates the morning hunt for homework and backpack and ensures the finished work is there when it's time to hand it in.

At the end of study time, it's inspection time. Ask yourself: Did my child put in the time and make good use of it, or did he sit there with arms folded? Did my child show a decent effort or whine while making paper airplanes? In rehabilitating a child with behavior problems, we focus in this area primarily on attitude rather than on completed work. Otherwise, we would find ourselves saying, "Get back in there until it's done!"

A child won't fail homework inspection just because the work is incomplete. If a child wants to keep working, that's fine, but the parent doesn't have to coerce the child to keep working until the homework is done. Many a parent has told me that homework *should* take an hour but that with all the arguing it ends up taking three hours. Our schedule eliminates the need to fight about homework all night. After the scheduled study time, we can consider the matter closed . . . until tomorrow. If a child puts in the time and effort and gets nowhere, the study expectations may be excessive; in that case, the matter should be discussed with the child's teacher. If a learning disability is suspected, that, too, may require testing and an Individualized Education Plan.

Remember, we can't expect perfect attitude right off the bat, but we want to reward children who are going in the right direction, behaviorally speaking. If a child fusses for ten minutes but then settles in and works for thirty, early on in the program that could be a pass. If a child tries to sneak away to use a cell phone, that is a different matter. Parents need to be vigilant during study time to make sure that children are not stealing rewards.

A word about cell phone use. Cell phone use is a reward, and as a reward, it can be denied if expectations are not met. A boy was seeing me for psychiatric problems, and his mother told me that her son would have a fit if she took away his cell phone. I learned that the phone was currently out in the car. I asked the mother to confiscate it, then and there. Explaining to the boy that the phone had been confiscated would cause less conflict than trying to wrestle it away while he was talking on it to his girlfriend.

Chapter 7 presented an example of a morning schedule. In the afternoon, a schedule might begin like this:

3:00	Arrive home. Put backpack on kitchen table.
3:00–3:10	Get a snack and clean up the kitchen after yourself.
3:10–4:10	Study time.
4:10	Inspection.
4:10–6:00	Free time with or without rewards, depending on whether inspection was passed. Once free time is over, the children are to pick up their play things and put away electronic gadgets.

A pass after homework earns free time for the next hour or two. During free time the child can watch television, play video games, or do whatever things the child is accustomed to doing. Even within this free time parents can certainly decide to limit the amount of time spent watching television or playing video games.

Other rewards will be designated, depending upon the age of the child. For younger children, the reward might include playing with certain toys; for older children, things like telephone and computer privileges. The reward might include using the swimming pool. Parents simply need to ask themselves what their child usually does in free time after school. Think about the "big ticket" items, the things that parents have paid for but that do not constitute the necessities of life. These things need to be looked at as the privileges they are.

What can children do if they have failed the inspection? First of all, no one is going to stop them from working on the homework they refused to do earlier. But now it's too late to get a pass. Holding fast to this rule quickly teaches kids that the world doesn't run on their time.

Failing an inspection does not necessarily mean that children are sent to their room. They are not automatically on time-out. The focus belongs on what they *cannot* do, namely, any of the previously defined rewards. They can do anything else. If, over time, you notice that your child consistently plays happily with action figures or on the trampoline after failing inspection, you might consider adding those activities as rewards in the "treasure box."

One reason rewards might not work is that there are too many rewards around to manage. Think: garage sale.

We asked earlier what kids can do if they fail inspection. Answer: anything that hasn't been identified as a reward. Maybe they can explore the backyard (unless you know that spells trouble). Thus, the punishment can even turn into a positive experience, since many children probably watch too much TV and play too many video games as it is. Young children may color. Older children can read. If, however, the child is an excellent reader who cares nothing for TV or video games and is only too happy to become absorbed in science fiction books, then those books are serving as a natural reward for the child. The books can be put on a bookshelf that is called "the library," and they can be checked out upon passing inspection.

For younger children who are primarily interested in toys, their favorite toys can be boxed up. The box needs to be kept in the parents' possession, and the toys must be handed out only if the child passes inspection. At cleanup time these toys are returned to the box. Other, less desirable toys can remain in the child's room, and the child can play with them even after failing inspection. Following a child around once he has failed inspection to make sure that he is miserable is not the point or the goal.

I explained above that we do not want the rewards to be taken away for days or weeks at a time, although there can be exceptions to this rule. Thus, for the purposes of our generic schedule, the day has been broken down into morning, school time, after school, and evening sections. If children put in their time on homework (I almost slipped and said, "If they have *done* all their homework"), then they will pass inspection and have full access to the rewards for the rest of the afternoon. Then comes evening.

9

When Evening Comes

At a certain time of day the toys are put away and older children are expected to be home from their friends' houses for the evening meal. The schedule should specify these expectations. One way of making these expectations clear on the schedule is to include them in the next block of time:

6:00–6:10	Pick up things used during free time. Be home from friends' houses.
6:10–6:40	Dinner. (Dessert is for people who eat dinner.) Take your own plate to the sink.

Of course, it will not always be possible to have dinner at the same time every day. However, consistency is a goal to shoot for, as it is for any kind of learning or exercise program. Perhaps your child can play a role in either setting the table or preparing the meal. This need not be an absolute expectation but can be an invitation to interact. What we *can* expect is for children to join the family at the dinner table and to behave in a civilized way during the meal. After dinner would be an ideal time for an adolescent to have a chore, such as wiping off the table, taking out the garbage, or feeding a pet. Even little ones can be assigned an after-dinner chore like carrying their plate to the sink or getting ready for a bath.

A Chore Schedule

In behavior rehab, consistent expectations are better than switching off chores between siblings. If you *want*, you can use a rotating chore chart that spells out which child has which job during a particular week. A potential problem is that kids will complain about whose turn it is and who didn't do a good job last time.

Parents may want to use the principles in this book for any and every child (and other people in their lives). But I usually recommend creating one schedule at a time, focusing on the most problematic child. I tell parents that they do not have to make a schedule for their other kids. If you want to, fine, but don't do it just to be fair to the problem child. Your children are different people and can be treated accordingly. Some problem children will say, "If I'm gonna have this schedule, then Missy is too." Missy's behavior is your business, not her brother's. You can reply (or just think), "Missy isn't the one who spit on the principal." If I were to make a Top Ten list of important life lessons, learning to mind one's own business would be in the top five.

Not using coercion doesn't mean that you are giving your problem child permission not to do his chore. The other children in the family will realize this when they learn that he isn't joining them to go to the movies. They may even be the ones who beg you to let him come along.

Even if it seems easier for you to take out the garbage than to risk having the child spill it, part of our project is to raise expectations. That might mean teaching new skills. Accidents will happen, and they are an opportunity for you to model patience. But if you won't have enough patience at the end of the day, it would be better to forget assigning garbage duty as a chore. Onward!

If you *can* have a consistent dinnertime, the schedule for immediately after dinner might read:

6:40–7:00   Take out recyclables. Wipe off table.
              Feed the rabbits.
7:00   Inspection.

For families whose dinnertime varies widely because of work schedules, I suggest the following: if dinner is later, it means more free time for the kids before dinner and less after. Once dinner is over, a specific *amount of time*, rather than a specific time by the clock, is given for the next order of business. The schedule can read:

End of dinner.   Within 20 minutes, take out
                   recyclables, wipe off table, feed
                   the rabbits.

Once a reasonable amount of time has been given for children to take care of their responsibilities, it is once again time for the parent to do an inspection. Note that it may have been only a couple of hours since the previous inspection. Children are given a fresh opportunity for success. Even if they failed the previous inspection, they can pass this one and perhaps be allowed some time with those same rewards that they failed to earn before. Some of those rewards may no longer be available, of course. If it's too dark to go outside, then that is not an option. It's up to the parent to decide.

7:00–8:00   Free time with or without rewards.

Time for Bed

After children pass the evening inspection, they are allowed access to the rewards for the next hour or so until it is time for the bedtime routine. This routine may include bathing or showering. One problem we run into is that we have come to the end of the day, and the child has no more rewards to work for. For this reason, if bath time is a problem in your house, then perhaps it should be moved up to the time right after dinner, especially for younger children. Instead of taking out the garbage, they are expected to take a bath, and if they pass, they can earn some fun activities for that evening. If they fail, either they do not earn those activities or perhaps they have to go to bed earlier.

Although bathing and showering in the morning works well for some families, it might be easier to have young children bathe in the early evening to avoid the hustle and bustle of the morning. Some children have an additional inspection after bath time, and if all went well—the towels got hung up, and there was no water on the floor—they can earn half an hour of reading in bed. Otherwise, they go to bed half an hour earlier.

8:00–8:30	Bath time. Hang up your towel. Brush teeth.
8:30	Inspection.
8:30–8:50	Passing inspection earns a story for little children or quiet play and bedtime at 8:50. A fail results in bedtime at 8:30.

For older kids, free time after dinner (with or without telephone or other devices, depending on the result of inspection) can extend further into the evening, especially if they can shower without prompting at the end of the day and put themselves to bed. In our house, we end the day with family prayers (which usually begin with great discussions about whatever the kids are wondering about). Then the little ones go to bed; the big ones read or may need to study a while longer before they go to sleep.

Working Parents

In single-parent households and in families with two working parents, modifications need to be made. If you must get home later than your children, remember that you can't expect what you cannot inspect. It doesn't matter if they show you the homework they've done. You still won't know what they were supposed to work on. It is usually not reasonable to expect teachers to be in daily communication with parents about assignments. Going online to a homework hotline is only more work for you. Again, it's supposed to be your kids' work, not your work.

If our concern is children who are having trouble in school because they aren't doing homework, the only way to address our concern is to monitor how the children are using their study time. For parents who get home an hour after their child, I recommend that homework and housework be switched in the schedule. When you arrive home, you won't know whether your child has put in an hour studying, but you can walk into the house and see whether the dishes have been put away or the garbage has been taken out and whether the house has been trashed.

3:00–3:20	Arrive home. Backpack on table. Hang up coat. Get snack and clean up afterward.
3:20–3:25	Put away dishes.
3:25–4:00	Mom arrives home.
4:00–4:10	Visit with Mom.
4:10–5:10	Study time.
5:10	Inspection.
5:10–6:10	Free time with or without rewards, depending on whether inspection was passed. Clean up stuff when free time is over.
6:10–6:40	Dinner.

There is a potential problem here. What if Mom arrives home to find that the dishes have not been put away and the house is a mess? This means a failed inspection and no rewards, but the children have already had free access to TV and other rewards. That is, they have been paid in advance of doing any work, so when you say, "No computer tonight," who cares? They can just wait until tomorrow after school when you aren't home. Now you are faced with putting little suitcase locks into the prongs of the TV electrical cord, and those locks don't come off until you are home and see that the dishes have been put away and the house is clean. That means also locking kids out of the computer and video games. There is no perfect solution for not monitoring kids who need to be monitored. The more time they are not monitored, the more likely they are to get into worse and worse trouble. When we are working to stop drug abuse in rehabilitation, for example, first and foremost that means limiting opportunities, which translates into increased monitoring.

Some parents need to use after-school care. If your child is actually doing the required studying after school at a relative's house or at "homework club" and has the good grades to prove it, you are lucky. Unless the person watching your child can take full responsibility for monitoring study time and making sure that it's well spent and passes inspection before free time starts, it may be best not to expect the child to study right after school. Maybe he can do some reading at his aunt's house, but I would recommend that you still expect some study time once you are home. It would be much easier not to, but the parent who wants behavioral change needs to practice being the one providing the structure. If you think your child has problems only at school, it's good to find out what happens when you place a few demands on him or her.

For a high school student who spends the afternoon at a relative's or at basketball practice and is home with you in the evening:

6:10–6:40   Dinner.
6:40–8:10   Study time.
8:10   Inspection.
8:10–9:30   Free time with or without phone, TV, computer or video games, depending on inspection results.
9:30–10:00 Wind down (no phone or electronics). Shower. Get ready for bed.
10:00   Lights out.

Some parents are heroic. In order to get their child on track, they will change their hours at work or take a leave of absence or even quit a job so they can be there when their child comes home from school. Not every parent can take these steps. Those parents who can, and do, deserve a hero's reward.

10

*Weekends, Holidays, and
Long-Term Rewards*

As relaxed and unscheduled as weekends tend to be, you
may feel that you do not want to use a behavioral schedule
on Saturday or Sunday—or on holidays, either. Before you
make this decision, however, ask yourself whether you truly
have *zero* expectations for your children on the weekends.
If you have any expectations at all for Saturday and Sunday,
these will require monitoring.

Children think up all kinds of fun activities for the weekend. Will they be allowed these activities without earning
them? And how will you know if they earned them or not?
You have to monitor! Once you are tuned into the benefits
of behavioral rehabilitation, you realize it makes no sense to
operate without it. Some kids don't need a written schedule,
weekends or any other time, but only because they already
have it down. They know when to work and they know when
to play. For kids who do need behavior modification, making
steady progress is more difficult if they have no structure on
weekends and then try to restart things Monday morning.

A weekend schedule doesn't mean bugle call at 6 a.m. If
your child is used to sleeping in until noon, you do not have
to change that, but you do have to be clear: Make the bed
and pick up your room before Honey Nut Cheerios and car-
toons or sporting events on TV. Complete chores before

spending the rest of the day playing with friends. And Mom or Dad will do a quick inspection before forking over ten dollars for a movie.

A variation on the inspection process might be useful on weekends when you don't want to keep a child indoors for hours because of a failed inspection. Instead of pass or fail being determined absolutely at a specified inspection time, the kids are told that *free time doesn't start* until they pass inspection. That way, you aren't committed to keeping them indoors all afternoon, but the more time they take to *do* the chores, the less time they have available for play. Just be sure they aren't playing on the computer when they are supposed to be working.

A weekend schedule might include specific chores and routines (hanging up towels after using them, for example, and putting dishes in the sink after a snack) as well as the requirement "Be home by dinner time."

If your children can't be trusted to be home for dinner, they can have friends over but they can't go anywhere until the day they earn your trust. Kids will ask how they can earn trust to be home on time without being allowed to go anywhere. The answer is that the person who can be trusted in small matters can be trusted in greater ones. By passing all their inspections at home, they will prove they are ready for bigger things.

The weekend evening schedule probably looks like the weekday evening one, give or take an hour (see Chapter 9).

Holidays away wreak havoc on schedules. Exercise schedules, diets, and behavior rehab schedules—all are disrupted. But parents who are serious about changing their children's behavior will have a plan ready and waiting for the holidays. That way, the children will know what to expect ahead of time, and the transition will be as smooth as possible. Even after a night in a motel, if kids dress and put away the rollaway bed *before* they turn on the room TV, it saves everybody grief. Holidays at home might just look like a string of Saturday schedules, minus some chores but with other ones included, like getting the house ready for company.

Assessing the Week

To the short-term, daily elements of the schedule we want to add some longer-term rewards or consequences. We continue to monitor the daily routine, and we also look at how the week goes as a whole. The pattern—expectation, inspection, reward—remains the same. Our expectation is that kids have a decent week. Toward the end of each week, families begin to consider plans for the weekend. Now those considerations ought to take into account how the week has gone because the weekend and its activities are a reward. The overall assessment of the week takes the place of the inspection.

If your children have had a good week, when the weekend rolls around, you will want to show them that you appreciate their efforts. The child who has accepted the schedule and has worked hard to pass inspections morning, afternoon, and evening should earn not only the usual rewards of the weekday but also "interest." The child should be acknowledged at week's end for having done a good job and should be rewarded with something good for that weekend. That doesn't mean spending money you don't have. It might mean allowing your child to attend a sleepover at a friend's house.

But shouldn't there be consequences for the children who have failed inspection all week? Don't those failed inspections indicate that they don't care about rewards? The consequence may be something as simple as requiring those children to stay home. They should still follow the weekend schedule, but passing inspections earns limited rewards: no going to the movies, no friends visiting.

The Family Meeting

The perfect way to accomplish this goal of connecting the week to the weekend is with a family meeting. At the end of the week, perhaps Friday over dinner, the children are given serious (but never insulting) feedback about how the week went. It also happens to be the time when the children make their desires known concerning the weekend. If your high school teen is accustomed to going to the football game Friday night, the family meeting can be on Thursday (always with the understanding that going out depends on passing all inspections Friday, also). Going out Friday might mean getting chores done earlier than usual. A child can always ask for an early inspection to increase free time. It's the late chores that don't work, just as you can pay your income tax *early*, but not *late*, without paying a penalty.

What's the best way to keep track of the week's progress? Some parents can do it by "feel." Others prefer to keep written notes of inspections passed versus inspections failed. The more challenging your child, the more important it is to keep a written account of inspections passed, so you can show visible evidence to the child (and yourself) that actions have consequences. One mother had the rehab schedule laminated. She used a dry erase marker to track passes and fails in a column right on the schedule; she wiped it clean at the start of a new week.

Fun weekends are the natural reward for a week of good effort. A child who has had a good week is going to learn that hard work pays off. But a kid who has been late getting to school several days might not earn certain privileges for that weekend. That child might miss out on going to a movie, and she is definitely not sleeping over at a friend's house or using the car.

There are times during the week when it's impossible to

enforce a consequence: the child skips toothbrushing after morning inspection has already been passed and everyone is heading out the door, or he disrespects you in public or refuses to take his medicine. Often there is no way to address the behavior on the spot. Of course if missing a dose of medicine would be life-threatening, rather than feeding the child's addiction to conflict, you might just boldly and decisively take the child to the doctor's office or the emergency room. If missing a dose of medicine is not life-threatening, you might let it go. But if there is any misbehavior due to the lack of medicine, whose fault would that be? The family meeting is a good time to let a child know that the miscellaneous transgressions, while they were overlooked at the time, can have an impact on the weekend. I hasten to add that forgiving a child may also be in order.

The weekly family meeting is a time for praise, a time to catch your child being good and to say "Thank you for trying." If a child had a rough Monday and Tuesday but pulled it together—even went above and beyond the rest of the week—there is still hope for doing something fun that weekend. We want to reward progress . . . within reason.

One family that I worked with did a pretty good job during the week of laying down the law. However, regardless of how the week went, they always wanted their daughter to be able to go to the dances and other school activities, thinking these would be good social experiences. Progress was made, but it was excruciatingly slow because their daughter seemed to know what her parents did not: she could avoid unpleasant tasks and still go to the dances as long as she behaved on Thursday and Friday.

Just as weekend privileges depend on how the week goes, longer-term rewards should be determined by how the month goes. For instance, if Barb behaves well for a couple of months, she might take all her friends to a ballgame and then attend a sleepover. Or if Travis keeps his grades up, he might be able to get his driver's license. Grades are a good measure for monitoring long-term progress.

Level Systems and Allowances

In a level system, the question is "What level of reward has the child earned?" A child earns points to reach a certain level. Each level has its own privileges. This system is commonly used in group homes. A child at the highest level might be allowed to go with supervisory staff to the neighborhood swim center on Saturdays. A child who has been violent might "lose his level" and have to stay home. Levels can be earned back by behaving the following week.

A star chart is a similar way of tracking who has been naughty and who has been nice. For good behavior young children earn a star on their chart, visual evidence of compliance or the lack thereof. Earn enough stars and you can cash them in. This is also known as a token economy.

Some parents have used level systems with their challenging kids to no avail. *A level system works only if it is the icing on the cake; that is, if it is used on top of a fully functional rehab schedule.* A level system may be needed for more difficult children (that's why such systems are used in group homes).

In a level system for difficult children, your behavior plan can use the family meeting to determine what privilege level a child earns, not just for the weekend but for the entire coming week. Passing 90 percent of the inspections during the week might earn gold status, which translates into all privileges being available for the following week. (The privileges are *available*, but inspections still must be passed as usual.) A pass rate of 80 to 90 percent would be silver. At a silver level, even when inspection is passed on Saturday morning or Monday after school, Travis can earn only a half hour of playing time on his Nintendo system. Other privileges, like music and TV, are still available, still there to motivate. We never want to remove all privileges ahead of time, or there will be no point in passing inspection. If a child passes fewer than 80 percent of his inspections, he earns bronze. He may still earn privileges, but favorite activities such as playing video games would be eliminated for the entire week, until the next family meeting.

If you want to give an allowance, a child could earn one or two dollars for each weekday he passes every inspection. At the weekly family meeting, he can get his paycheck: anywhere from zero to five or ten dollars.

Expectations or Consequences

If there's one thing families have in common, it's that their weekends vary greatly. Don't let that stop you from using a schedule. If you always go to the lake on weekends in the summer, then go, but Daniel doesn't have to be allowed to swim or water ski. If you love to go out to dinner, you can still go, but pack a PB&J sandwich for the misbehaving child. If the attitude starts on the way to the restaurant, he can drink water instead of Sprite. Once you learn the language of behavior modification, you can begin to use your imagination.

If any of this sounds mean spirited, understand that behavior modification is designed to create a new way of interacting between parent and child that will take the place of the emotionally—and certainly the physically—abusive relationship that has been established by past behaviors (on the part of both parents and child).

There is some value in letting a child spoil everyone's good time. If you are never willing to let this happen, it teaches children they can get away with anything. One mother told her badly behaved daughter that she couldn't go see *Shrek* at the theater, but then Mom decided that *she* wanted to see the movie, and by gum, she wasn't going to suffer, so they went anyway.

Missing a movie, or turning around and coming home from a restaurant or the state fair, is a small price to pay to teach a child that you mean business. Threats without follow-through are worse than useless: they teach kids that grown-ups don't follow through. Allowing the whole family to suffer together is part of being a family. If everyone is mad at the one who spoiled everything, that is fair enough.

Sometimes parents are only too happy to have the child disappear for a few hours for a birthday party. They will even feel sorry for the child who is having the birthday party, and so they let their undeserving child attend. I think this is a mistake. The birthday child will certainly not be traumatized for life if one fewer kid shows up, and the other parents ought to understand.

Sports and Jobs

Some parents let their children play soccer games on the weekend, no matter what. Parents need to ask themselves whether soccer is a reward or an expectation for their child. If they decide it is an expectation, then the child clearly will be going to that soccer game regardless of what kind of week it was. However, playing sports usually serves as a reward for children. I recommend that a child who has just had the week from hell not be allowed to play.

One idea that helps in regard to sports is that a child who fails afternoon inspection during the week might miss practice that day. That child needs to be informed that missing practice is letting the team down and that the situation cannot continue. If the child misses a total of three practices or games based on bad behavior, the child can no longer be on the team simply because unreliability has a negative impact on the other team members as well as on the coach.

It may be difficult to decide whether an activity is more reward or expectation. This question needs to be considered for things like jobs, Little League Baseball, Scouts, and piano lessons. If it's something the child wants, then it is partly a reward. If it's something the child might not choose (e.g., piano lessons), then the lessons are an expectation. The lessons should be treated like an extension of school, and practicing should be treated like homework.

But what if a child is not doing well in school and not behaving well at home? One has to wonder about adding piano as an expectation for a child who is not meeting what are arguably more basic expectations. Similarly, a teenager who is not meeting basic academic and household expectations probably has no business holding down a job. It is out of order. For problematic kids, the times before, during, and after work provide an opportunity to do unhealthy, prohibited things such as experiment with drugs. One patient of mine who had an eating disorder was able to leave her job for a few minutes and go to a nearby drugstore to buy laxatives. The job put her in proximity to the drugstore and gave her an opportunity that she would not otherwise have had.

Another trap parents get caught in is thinking that it is good for the child's socialization skills to be on a sports team. First, I would point out that this kind of parental thinking turns the sport into an expectation rather than a reward for the child. Such children eventually will not want to play sports, and a sport becomes one more thing to argue about. Sports certainly are an excellent avenue for teaching social skills. But if a child is disrespectful to parents and siblings and is being allowed to play sports in order to become socialized, there is something wrong with the picture.

As I said earlier, children usually show their worst behavior to their parents, but if it continues, over time it will begin to leak out into school . . . and into sports as well. Children who behave poorly for their parents will eventually behave poorly for their coach and will not be team players. Charity and good behavior begin at home. Once children learn to behave well in their own family, they are in a much better position to enjoy the responsibilities that go along with athletics. *Kids who are praised and given privileges for their athletic prowess while being allowed to get away with antisocial behavior are a danger to society.*

11

Troubleshooting

*Complaining, Disrespectful,
Out-of-Control Behavior.*

If your computer doesn't work when you turn it on, you will probably look for the troubleshooting chapter in the computer manual. The first entry in the troubleshooting section will ask, "Is the computer plugged in?"

Until kids are motivated by their own desire for future success, parents can plug into natural rewards as their power source. Negative consequences provide a backup, but we hope our kids grow up *wanting to do the right thing* rather than fearing punishment for doing the wrong thing. The schedule embodies the hope that kids will be motivated by their own desire for future success—that is the spirit behind the schedule.

Make no mistake: it is possible to have a complete behavioral system in place and then completely sabotage it with too much talking. Parents must have a sense of whether their child perceives them as encouraging or controlling. The only way to establish that you are not controlling is to allow kids to fail. And you must realize that their failure is not a reflection on you. Once kids trust that a parent will respect their freedom, they will be able to focus, first on the reward and eventually on wanting to please the parent who has won their trust and respect.

Some parents very quickly gain an insight into the spirit of the schedule. They understand it and believe that they can implement it without actually writing up a schedule. Usually what happens is that things work out OK for a short period of time, but then everybody falls back into the old habits. *Write up the schedule.*

Parents have a tendency to assume that it is the child's responsibility to make sure the schedule is kept in good working order. I ask parents to go home and type up a final draft of the schedule we have discussed, so we can review it again before they present it to the child. Many parents come back with a schedule showing what the child is supposed to do, but somehow the inspection times have disappeared! Sometimes this is an unconscious error on the parents' part, and they quickly see the need to fix it. Sometimes, however, parents say that they have consciously omitted the inspection because it is *a given* that there will be an inspection after the work is done and before the play begins. In my experience, remembering to do an inspection is anything but a given. Parents need the firm commitment of a written time. Unless the parent is firmly committed to doing an inspection, the system quickly deteriorates into a situation where the child is once again watching TV and the parent is asking the child, "Did you clean your room? Did you work on your homework?" The parent needs to know the answer to those questions before the television goes on. Otherwise, the new system is really just the old system all over again.

Consider the rough draft shown here, which was written by one mother for her nine-year-old son. She did a pretty nice job, but there are some problems. Failing the morning inspection means "No TV all day." But in the afternoon, a pass earns TV. How can her child earn TV in the afternoon if he has already lost it for the entire day? We fixed that: TV does not appear at all in the morning schedule, but TV can be earned in the afternoon. The only consequence in the

Schedule

Weekdays
1. 6:30–7 a.m. Get up, dress, make bed, brush teeth & hair
2. Inspection: 7 a.m. Put shoes on / get backpack in car
3. Reward—
   P — Warm breakfast 7–7:30 a.m.
   F — Cold cereal (F)
   F — No TV all day (F)

After School
1. Take shoes off, wash hands, snack, discuss day
2. Homework 30 minutes
3. Inspection
   P — Go outside & play or watch TV or go to park
   F — Do housework, matching socks, cleaning bathroom, cleaning closets, drawers

Dinner
1. Wash hands, help with dinner, set table
2. Eat dinner; if picky eater, cold dinner or sandwich
3. Put dishes in dishwasher, clean table
4. Take a shower, brush teeth & hair
5. Inspection
6. Free time
   P — Go outside & play, watch cable; lights out 8:30 p.m.
   F — Go to bed at 6:30; read until 7:30 p.m. — lights out

Weekends
Shopping
Eating out
Birthday parties
Basketball game
Kings game

morning is cold cereal. That may not seem like much, but kids are affected at a psychological level just knowing that they lost something (unless they get their own rewards in provoking their parent).

Another problem with the schedule is that in the afternoon the times of day have disappeared. This mother worked, and it turned out that her child had homework club after school. Mom could not monitor study time, and the homework was not getting done. I recommended that her child be expected to do half an hour of homework when the family arrived home at 5:00. If homework has already (supposedly) been done, then the child could spend the half hour reading. Mother and child needed the experience of Mom being the one in charge, not the people at homework club. When the boy's reputation and grades begin to reflect that he truly does all his homework at the club, the schedule can be modified.

There is another problem with this schedule. If the boy fails the homework inspection, he is supposed to do housework. But why would he do housework if he won't do homework? Mom will be forced to badger him or give up. If he fails to study, he should just *lose the rewards*.

I worked with one family on a behavior plan for their daughter who had been hospitalized for out-of-control behavior. Things had been going well for the first couple of months after hospitalization when I received a call from the mother saying that she did not know what had happened. The system had been working well, but now she could no longer get her daughter to do the things she was supposed to do. I had to remind her of the spirit of the schedule: She was not supposed to *get* her daughter to do anything. She was only supposed to check that the things had been done that were supposed to have been done. Over the course of a couple of months, the system had deteriorated into the mother trying to force the girl to take care of her obligations. As soon as this happened, the girl fell back onto her old habit of saying no.

The power source that we should use is the child's natural inclination toward fun. However, as long as the *other* power source is still plugged in—namely, the parent's tendency to coerce the child—the system will be too full of static for the child to see clearly what needs to be done to achieve happiness.

For these reasons, a schedule never says that it is time for the parent to argue with the child. But what about children who pick fights with their parents?

Two Types of Conflict

There are two major types of conflict—call them Type One and Type Two. Conflict Type One is generated by the parent, Type Two by the child. In each case, parents want one thing, and the child wants another. In conflict Type One, a parent insists that an unwilling child do something. Thus it is the parent who actually starts the conflict. In conflict Type Two, a child wants something. The child may want to play a video game; the child may want (negative) attention; the child may want to exert control over the parent's emotions.

We can eliminate the first kind of conflict by not fighting with kids to make them work. *We are not going to cause conflict ourselves.* That decision goes incredibly far toward decreasing stress in the family system and promoting better behavior. An ounce of promoting good behavior is worth at least a pound of dealing with bad.

Looking back at the system of vicious cycles, we see the word *conflict*. When we began, conflict was just conflict. It was as unpredictable as it was nasty. Now we know that there are two kinds of conflict. Now that we as parents are not going to start the conflict, we can easily predict when a child will start a conflict: at precisely 5:10 p.m., when the child fails homework inspection and can't watch TV.

It is the child, not us, who causes the second kind of conflict. In conflict Type Two, the child who has refused to do chores now wants something from the parent and is antagonizing the parent (or a sibling) to get that something. The same kid who claims not to care about rewards is often the one who has parents walking around on eggshells. That same child can go ballistic when a reward is taken away. *Let us bury forever the idea that rewards don't matter.*

Children come into this world naturally equipped with certain behavioral modification skills: they cry until they get what they want. That is how they modify the behavior of their parents. When older children are angry about not getting something they want, they generally choose one of three behaviors: complaining, showing disrespect, or being out of control.

The Child Who Complains

A child's complaints or gripes about having failed an inspection present an opportunity for the parent. If children truly don't understand why they didn't pass inspection, then the reason can be explained. More likely, kids know exactly why they didn't pass inspection, and they're simply complaining about not getting their way. In this case, parents need to be confident that they have been more than fair with the child: they have not asked anything excessive, they have not coerced, and the punishment has not been excessive.

If justice means giving to others their due, it also means that we *don't* have to give to others what is *not* due them. In this case, children are not always due an explanation for every decision a parent makes. A little explanation can be helpful, as long as that's the end of it, and it's not just a prelude to an argument. Overexplaining is a major pitfall in training children. When the child complains that Mom or Dad is not being fair, the parent should not get hooked into explaining unnecessarily. Parents have to make many decisions in the course of a day, and they have no obligation to explain every decision to a disgruntled child who is whining, "Why? I wanna know why!"

To decide whether an explanation is appropriate, consider what would happen if you just gave in and gave your children whatever they wanted. Would they still care about why you said no at first? Consider telling your children that you will explain your reasons at a later time; for the moment, you want them to accept your decision. By all means explain yourself later. More than likely you will discover that the children did not really *want* an explanation of how you were thinking. They simply wanted to get their way. It is okay for kids to question authority, but there is a time and a place for it.

Kids learn just what to say to get their parents' attention. If calling Mom a bozo gets no response, the word *bozo* may not get used again. But if saying "You never listen to me!" gets Mom's attention, you can bet it will be used again. Kids learn what buttons to push. Like a good fisherman, they learn what bait works to hook a parent. Parents are more likely to take the bait if they have already been provoked by the child's refusal to do a chore. When a grown-up is provoked, some kids will behave—and others will smell blood. These children are the ones addicted to conflict. Once parents have overcome the voice inside their own head that tells them they have to demand obedience, kids will realize that it's not their parents who have the problem.

On an old game show, *The Newlywed Game,* the host was always baiting the couples to argue with each other. You could say it was the original reality TV show. He would cause them to argue, and then he would ask them, "Who's right?" And the couple would argue some more.

Kids use the same technique when they don't get what they want. They know exactly which phrases to use to bait their parents. *The parent who is not already upset with a child's disobedience will see clearly what is happening:*

- "It's not fair!"
- "How come Bobby gets to?"
- "You're not my real dad!"
- "How come you never listen?"
- "You lied to me!"
- "I hate you."

- "Why?"
- "Why not?"
- "Why me?"

To my ear, all of this sounds like complaining. *If children can keep you talking long enough, they may get what they want. If they don't get what they want, they may keep complaining because they are addicted to the hidden reward: making you angry.* Your getting angry will only feed into this problem. Continuing to respond to your child as if the conversation you are having is rational will only prolong the agony.

What if the child says, "But you lied to me! You said I could!" and the father responds angrily, "You tell me! Did you clean your room like you were supposed to?" What's happened here is that the father has taken the bait and is essentially asking the child to respond with something like, "But please! I'm *saying* 'please'!" Now is not the time to explain that saying "please" doesn't get you everything you want. Besides, kids already know that.

Complaining (and responding to it) is not the same thing as having a real conversation. It's a game, a dance. It's like two children saying to each other:

"I did not!"
"You did too!"
"Did not!"
"Did too!"

Parents have to learn to tolerate the fact that their children will not always be happy and that ultimately some good can come from the suffering that the child experiences. Frustration builds frustration tolerance. Knowing that the schedule is fair will help prevent parents from becoming defensive with a child who is unhappy with them.

Try not to get angry with a child who is complaining about not earning a reward. And if you do explain yourself and your kid snaps, "Okay, okay, I *get* it!" please don't start commenting on her rude tone. Just let that be the end of it. If a child's tone of voice says, "It's *not* okay and I *don't* get it," it is very tempting, but treacherous, to launch into a more satisfactory explanation or to correct the child for having a rude tone. If a child walks away saying, "Gosh you're mean!" let it go. The child has dropped the subject and is walking away. Sure, the child has a ways to go toward learning respect. But Rome wasn't built in a day. If a child is disappointed and Mom in turn is upset by the child's disappointment, Mom runs two risks: first, of overexplaining, and second, of losing her temper.

When a parent complains that the child wants the last word, I know that the parent must want the last word. Demanding that a child give you the last word teaches that the last word must be worth fighting for. (If the child is being clearly disrespectful, that is another matter.) Teach kids that having the last word is not important. The best way to do this is by example.

Instead of responding directly to the griping, realize that besides wanting what they want, kids also want to voice their displeasure. They need to be able to do so without getting into trouble for it. If an unhappy child was griping about not earning time with the video game, I used to tell parents to simply ignore the complaints. My intention was to emphasize that I didn't want the parent getting sucked into another conflict. I wanted the parent to set an example that it is okay to give another person the last word.

These days I think there should be another step before ignoring the griping child. Ignore the specific gripe, but empathize with him. Say in so many words, "I understand how you feel about not being able to play on the computer." Then encourage the child by reminding him that there are other opportunities to earn the reward in the future, which might be later in the same evening. A kind word turneth away wrath, so ignore the complaint per se and respond, "Hang in there."

Often when people are complaining about their situation, they don't need others to explain or solve their problems for them; they just need to be understood. When this system is applied at its best, parents begin to emulate those top-notch adults who meet an angry child, not with anger or indignation, but with compassion. And because of the short-term nature of the schedule, if children complain about failing inspection, parents *can* be understanding: "Hang in there. I know you're mad, but it's only an hour and a half until you can pass your next inspection and then you can call Jenny."

When a child is complaining, you want to prevent a blowup if you can, but not by giving in. When children complain, it presents an opportunity to model what one should do when being provoked, teased, or bullied. I teach kids four techniques to use when being bullied. Parents can use these four techniques and teach their kids at the same time:

1. Change the subject. When a child complains, act like you didn't hear the complaint and say something like, "Would you look at that? I think it's going to rain."
2. Use humor. If a kid says, "You never let me do anything!" say: "I think I did . . . yes, it was about two years ago, I'm sure of it!"
3. Agree: "It's true, life doesn't seem fair sometimes."
4. React (but don't overreact) to a verbal jab with honesty: "It hurts my feelings when you say that."

Sometimes getting physically closer to a child, going on one knee to be at her level or lightly touching her on the shoulder, can defuse things. Kids want to be heard. Say, "I hear you."

If you sense that any interaction or explanation (other than giving in) is going to make the child angrier, then it is time to ignore the complaining, even walk away.

But what if your child keeps pestering you? It's time to set a limit. It's time to let the child know in no uncertain terms that the conversation is over. Once you do that, if the child says anything more, that equals disrespect.

The Child Who Is Disrespectful

Parents often ask me what they can say to their angry kid, as if finding the right words would solve the problem. You don't need a list of clever one-liners. Even if you had one, it wouldn't work. Sometimes the truth fits best. Tell your child, "I don't know what else to say." And, finally, say, "I'm done talking about it." Anyone who continues to pester after you have made it clear that you are finished talking has crossed a line. In the workplace, it is called harassment and it is against the law. At home, it is called disrespect and it cannot be tolerated.

When children are merely complaining, ideally they are met with empathy. If a child crosses the line and the griping becomes disrespect, the parent can no longer avoid confronting the child with the confident authority you have as a parent. Once you have said that the topic is closed, any more complaining, any more asking "Why not?" constitutes disrespect. Once a parent has said, "That's my final word on the subject," it doesn't mean the parent must now be silent. It means the parent needs to set a limit.

A limit is a boundary, a border that, when crossed, means the child is "not in Kansas anymore." When people act outside the limits of the law, they forfeit their rights. Setting a clear limit means letting children know exactly how close they are to being banished. I know of no better limit than three warnings before a child is sent to his or her bedroom. (If your child won't go to the bedroom when told to, read on. You need this book more than other parents.)

Who decides when the line is crossed? That is completely up to the parent. And it might change, depending upon your mood. Some days, you may feel like discussing why God gave parents authority over children. But if you let your children know that you have had a hard day, they can learn that means less leeway for griping.

Once parents have said they have finished the discussion, the next words out of Mom or Dad's mouth should *not* be, "I *said* I was finished talking!" That is still talking.

Sound the first warning *after* you are slightly annoyed but *before* you are really angry. I like letting kids know they are about to cross the border by asking, "Do I need to start counting?" Another way to clearly show that a limit is being set is by saying "No, and *don't* ask again!" With those words, you are making it as plain as possible that you are serious. A countdown has begun.

Parents who joke around all the time need to work on not confusing their child by joking around. Let the child know absolutely by your posture and your tone of voice that if there is any more disrespect, the child will officially receive one warning: "That's one." A low growl works well. Even shouting "That's one!" is better than getting sucked back into telling the child again and again, "I told you no. Now stop," or explaining how you "are too" being fair, or saying something hurtful. The child is about to learn (if it hasn't been explained ahead of time) that if he needs to be told, "That's one . . . that's two . . . that's three," there is going to be a consequence. Three warnings. Not fifty. Remember that we want to cut down on the amount of correcting we do in order to decrease stress.

Don't give a mini lecture in between counts, such as this one: "That's one, little lady! You're really headed for trouble now! I'd think you would be more grateful after I took you to McDonald's yesterday." That is just the old way with three numbers tacked on. It will provoke your child to respond— and probably not politely.

Saying "That's one" should be followed by silence. If the child mumbles but is quieting down, leave it alone. Give your child an opportunity to wind down. But if plain disrespect continues after one warning, the child should be quickly told, "That's two." If parents use this system consistently, kids will eventually be able to stop themselves after Mom or Dad says, "That's one." It trains their brains.

By using three warnings, we are providing children with a runway where they can slow themselves and then stop. However, the runway does not go on forever. If kids get to three, the most common consequence is that they will be told to go to their room. Time to take a chill, also known as time-out.

Time-out provides a respite for children, something they're not always able to provide for themselves. We all need breaks from heated situations, and we, as adults, learn when we need to walk away from a situation. If we cannot leave the room, we learn at least to mentally distance ourselves from the situation. Many children have not yet learned this self-control. In this sense, time-out is not so much a punishment as an opportunity to teach children a skill they will use all their lives.

Time-out is a negative consequence in the sense that it deprives the child of the family's company. Time-out means time out from social interaction. It tells the child, "If you are going to behave that way, you cannot be with the rest of the family."

Time-out is best done in the child's or teenager's bedroom or some other room away from people. Children who have to take time-out in a corner are very tempted to continue to engage in social interaction with the parent by tapping their feet or tapping the walls, turning around and sticking out their tongue, and so on. Have them go to their room but don't insist they sit on their bed. Time-out is already a power struggle; there is no need to complicate it by insisting kids sit on their bed. Many parents think that their child should not be able to play with anything when on time-out. Of course, kids should not be allowed access to anything they failed to earn. No TV or video games in the bedroom. But it's okay for them to draw or play with a toy that is not off-limits. In this way, kids learn to distract themselves from being angry and learn how to calm down.

One mother brought in a tape recording of how time-out went at home. On the tape, I could hear her young boy shouting, and periodically I could hear her voice as she went into the room, calmly telling him to quiet down, to which he responded with increased volume and profanity. Children need to learn that time-out is not an opportunity for them to suck the parent back into a tug-of-war. Do not enter the room or further engage your child unless you fear for his or her safety.

Clarify how long the time-out is to last and make it clear to the child that the timer does not get set until the child is in the room and quiet. This puts the ball in the child's court. One minute for every year is a good rule of thumb: five minutes for a five-year-old, ten minutes for a ten-year-old. Ten minutes may even be long enough for most teenagers' limbic systems to cool down.

If a kid wants to go in and out of the room and shout, I ask parents not to respond. The time will not start on the clock until the child is in the room and quiet. If the child is quiet for two minutes and then begins to scream and kick the walls, time starts over again when he is quiet. This method saves you from adding ten more minutes every time the child mouths off. Adding time is a good way to end up with a five-hour time-out, which isn't feasible.

What we are asking for is five or ten straight minutes of calm behavior. Children who have spent ten minutes shouting are going to come out of time-out in worse shape than when they went in. Some kids refuse to go to their room altogether. That is a very serious problem that we will address shortly.

The three-warnings system is for a child who is acting obnoxiously or disrespectfully to you or anyone in the family, and it can be used any time of day. If you say, "That's one," and the child makes an effort to pull it together but does something obnoxious fifteen minutes later, you will probably want to start with one again.

Disrespecting siblings can also earn one warning. What if Joey insists that Nicole started it? You are the parent, you are the boss, and you have to start somewhere. Remind Joey that he has received only one warning and that you have your eye on Nicole for any false moves. All Joey has to do is behave for the next few minutes and the one warning will be forgotten. But if he protests vehemently because he won't tolerate having one false warning on his pure conscience, it tells you he is guilty. And here is a subtle but important point: Joey can be told that if he doesn't stop protesting he will earn a second warning.

Depending on the situation, bad language might warrant an automatic time-out, a warning, or just ignoring. Another method is to charge a quarter for profanity or for blatant rudeness toward parents or siblings. But if you end up feeling like you're charging too many quarters or giving too many time-outs, you need to do more ignoring of snide comments. Remember: Pay more attention to good behavior than to bad.

The three warnings are *not* meant to be used as threats to coerce a child to do some task. Do not say anything like "You better clean your room *now*, and that's *one*!" That's what inspection time is for. The reason we use an inspection time is to teach kids lessons about self-motivation that last a lifetime. Warnings and time-outs are used only when things have gone too far. (If you don't pay your income tax on time, the IRS is not going to say "That's one warning!" It is going to fine you!)

Taking a time-out is not the same thing as failing an inspection. If a child takes a time-out, all is forgiven, and he can still pass his next inspection. Refusing to take a time-out is a different matter. For small children who are showing an unwillingness to take time-out, I recommend telling them that you are going to count to ten, and if they are not in the room by ten, they are going be picked up and put into the room. If a small child refuses to stay in the room, there is no problem with redepositing him in the room and holding the door shut.

Using your greater strength in this situation is completely different from forcing a child to do a chore. In the real world, we do not force people to work—that is slavery—but if someone was in your house acting obnoxiously and refusing to leave, force might be called for. Foster parents can feel in a bind if they have been told not to put hands on a child. They are afraid of being accused of child abuse. But not teaching kids about limits is another kind of abuse. If they really mean to never lay hands on a child, foster parents need immediate backup from their agency simply to enforce time-out, not to mention handling dangerous behaviors.

Let's be clear: *picking a child up is a very different matter from hitting or slapping a child, which teaches kids to hit. We are not sparing the rod, we are subtilizing it.*

Refusing to Take Time-Out

What if a child refuses to take time-out or doesn't take it in a reasonable amount of time and is too big to be picked up? Defiance on this scale is getting close to the out-of-control behavior covered in the next section of this chapter. If a kid is not acting in a violent way but is refusing to go to her room, there are short-term and long-term consequences. The consequences are already built right into the schedule.

For example, if Jackie is angry because she failed the homework inspection, she should be encouraged to hang in there. If she is really serious about wanting to use the phone, as it now appears she is, she can wait a couple of hours, have dinner with the family, do her chore. She will pass evening inspection and be allowed to use the phone.

If she continues to complain, instead of telling her it's her own fault, Mom can change the subject and talk about what's for dinner. But if Jackie won't let it go, it's time to say, "That's one warning!" Bad language? That's two. If Jackie exhales in frustration, Mom can start making dinner. But if Jackie pops off again, that's three, and she is told to go to her room. Only she won't go. Go make dinner. Jackie probably won't even want to join you at dinner. (You might let her eat toast.) If she's mad enough, she won't be back on task to do her after-dinner chore. Therefore, the natural outcome of her refusal to take a simple time-out: she will fail the evening inspection and still not be permitted to use the phone. Even were she to do her chore, her attitude has clearly not been good. Recall our three essential elements of setting clear expectations:

1. *Quality.* How good is good enough? The standard you use should relate to the child's age and ability.
2. *Attitude.* A decent attitude is a prerequisite.
3. *Timeliness.* Set a deadline for when the task should be completed.

The attitude clause means that attitude counts when doing chores, but it doesn't mean that attitude doesn't count the rest of the time. There is never a time when children can do anything they please without consequences. Refusing to take time-out is a big mark against attitude. A child could fail an inspection by virtue of bad attitude alone. Still, when kids refuse time-out in the afternoon, you may want to use a carrot to get them back on track in time for evening chores. Refusing time-out in the afternoon might mean no telephone in the evening, but if Jackie pulls it together, has dinner, and does her evening chores, she could still earn half an hour of TV or be permitted to use her iPod.

Similarly, if kids refuse time-out in the evening, we don't want to start out the next morning expecting them to take the time-out. We want them to start the day with a clean slate. But there can be a reckoning come the weekend. The long-term consequence of refusing to take time-out might be: "This weekend there will be no movies, no sleepovers, and you will be sitting on the bench during your baseball game."

Let us say an eight-year-old child has refused time-out earlier but has now really pulled it together in the hope of passing the next inspection. Early on in rehab, that child might be praised for passing inspection but told, "There is just the small matter of an eight-minute time-out, and then you're free to enjoy watching the play-offs and possibly even salvage your weekend." Later in the process it no longer makes sense to keep allowing a child to pass inspections when he or she has refused to take time-out.

What if you are out in public when your child earns a time-out? There are no easy answers. Maybe you can use the car for time-out *if you keep watch out of the corner of your eye, and if it's not a hundred degrees out, and if the car keys are safely in your pocket, and so on.* You might just have to come home. Good behavior begins at home. Home is where the real practicing takes place. Kids who are super well-behaved at home usually don't suddenly become out of control in public.

If a child is supposed to be on time-out but has commandeered the PlayStation, take away the PlayStation. If the child is too big and you are afraid of getting hurt, bide your time. The situation may currently be out of control (see the next section in this chapter). The entire rehabilitation program is based on parents being in control of rewards. If use of the PlayStation can't be controlled, maybe the PlayStation shouldn't be in the house when your child wakes up the next morning. And the weekend plans—or lack thereof—should reflect his egregious behavior.

If you know your child is going to throw things when he is put in the bedroom, remove ahead of time anything you don't want thrown or broken. If your child will break the window, or sneak out of it, board it up. Does that sound absurd? What is absurd is a child who will break a window for being put on time-out.

If Maddy comes to the table with a nasty disposition, spoiling for a fight, and it bothers you immediately because your patience is worn thin and you know where the situation is headed, don't wait. Set a limit early. Calmly say, "I see what you're doing and I'm not going to put up with it." And if she responds with a nasty growl, you say, "That's one!" If, however, you are in a pleasant mood and are not stressed out (as many parents are at the end of the day), instead of immediately issuing the first warning, feel free to ask Maddy what is wrong or whether she would like to talk about anything. Maybe she'll talk it out. Or maybe you will still end up saying, "That's one." And if you get to three and she has locked herself in the bathroom, be sure you can easily open the lock. And once she's in her bedroom, if she begins throwing the pictures from her wall against the door, try not to yell. Instead, recognize that you should have removed those pictures before the time-out began, and tell her "Good night" even if it's only 6:30 in the evening. And next time, consider setting a limit earlier rather than later.

If you get kicked while putting your child on time-out, now is not the time to get into a discussion about why kicking is naughty—it's time to get out of the room! For something as outrageous as a kick in the face, your child can stay in there for an hour or two—or at least until you are sure you aren't going to hurt him. If it's after 6 p.m., maybe he can stay in there for the rest of the night. And if that doesn't seem like enough punishment, remember your family meeting on Friday and your control over weekend plans. Don't forget how angry and frustrated you were during the earlier time-out episode—even if, during the family meeting your child looks at you with big, hopeful eyes and asks about going to a birthday party.

So far in this chapter we have defined what we mean by complaining and disrespectful behaviors and discussed how to react to them in a way that will change your child's pattern of behavior. Now it's time to discuss out-of-control behavior. "Out of control" does not mean a screaming fit. The solution for a screaming fit is that time-out starts when the fit stops. Try not to worry too much what the neighbors think. If Child Protective Services shows up, let them see that you have food in your cupboards, promise to clean the top of your refrigerator, and show them this book.

Being Out of Control

Parents have to judge for themselves when a situation has gotten out of control. Some fires we can put out. But what if a fire is getting bigger instead of smaller? Please don't be afraid to call for help. Kids have crossed a serious line if they injure themselves or others, or if there is a credible threat that they will do so. Help is needed in these situations. Similarly, serious property damage calls for emergency action. If it can be predicted that a child will respond in a way that is dangerous, parents need to have an emergency plan.

The emergency plan can be calling a neighbor or relative over to the house, as long as the neighbor or relative's presence has the effect of getting the child's behavior under control. But if a child is engaging in serious property destruction, physical aggression toward others, or self-injury, it may be time to take your child to the nearest emergency room.

If you can't transport your child safely, call 911. If the police refuse to take your child because the child has calmed down by the time they arrive, perhaps your objective has already been achieved: the child is no longer dangerous. The officers will want you to take it from here. You might explain to them that the problem started when your child refused to take time-out and that before they leave you would still like your daughter to go to her room. With officers there, she will probably go. If instead of starting the time-out you want your child to be evaluated in a professional, psychiatric setting, it is up to you to make that happen. While the police are still with you is the time to get your child in the car yourself. If your child assaults you as you're walking to the car, the police may take a renewed interest.

No parents *want* their child to be hospitalized or to be placed in juvenile hall. But ask yourself, Who's really choosing that option, you or your child? If those services aren't warranted, don't send your child there. But if the situation calls for help and instead you give in to your child's demands, you are not helping in any way. You may in fact be reinforcing dangerous behavior.

I realize that some parents feel that psychiatric hospitalization should be avoided at all costs. They feel that it represents a failure on their part. I see it differently. I see psychiatric hospitals and emergency rooms, and even juvenile hall, as supports to parents who are raising children in a toxic day and age.

Some parents think that because they have called the police a time or two they have already used the system I am describing in this book. In reality they have only handled emergencies without having learned how to prevent them. Some parents will object and say that their child seems to *like* being in the hospital. I look at it this way: if there is a fire, you call for a firefighter. You wouldn't hesitate just because a certain firefighter seemed to actually enjoy fighting fires. If a kid needs to be hospitalized, everything else is secondary. Kids may like hospitals because in the hospital there is no conflict, no coercion. If a kid is hospitalized during the course of a behavior rehab program, the plan doesn't go away. It starts again the moment the child leaves the hospital. In fact it never stopped, since the hospital was a contingency of the plan from the beginning.

All along, we have been trying to increase the odds in favor of the child making a good choice. We have given the child many opportunities to make the right choice:

- First, the child can choose to do what has been clearly spelled out as expectations. If the child does not fulfill the expectations, he can choose to accept the consequences.
- If the child complains about the consequences, another choice exists: to accept the parent's empathic response "Hang in there." Or, at the least, the child can choose to respect the parent's decision to stop arguing.
- If the child grows disrespectful with the parent, yet another choice the child can make is to stop being disrespectful once the parent has given one warning.
- Or he can choose to go to the bedroom after receiving three warnings.

By setting the intervals between rewards only a couple of hours apart, we are trying to increase the likelihood that the child will accept the consequences now in order to be able to earn the rewards after a relatively short time. If, however, a child makes the wrong choice all the way down the line, or quickly goes all the way to threats of suicide or violence or property destruction, take it seriously. Even if you think the child is bluffing or doing it for attention, take it seriously and deal with it seriously, and don't stop until you've done your best to get your kid in a safe, structured environment. Do not bluff. If things seem dangerous, the time for reasonable chitchat is long past.

If your child is dangerous, it is time to take control. You may save a life. If the child was bluffing, you have taught him that you will always err on the side of safety. If you really don't think the child needs hospitalization, still keep a close watch. And later on, when the same child asks to spend the night at a friend's, the answer is "No, not while you may be suicidal." We want to be sure kids know that threats of suicide do not help them to gain privileges. On the contrary.

If a child runs away from home, it should be reported immediately to the authorities. But some kids are in the habit of running off when they are angry. That kind of running away is usually more of a pain than anything else. You have to make a judgment call. If you think your teen will return, you might have to wait it out. If you know whose house the teen ran to, call that parent. If you don't want your child at that house, tell the parent your child is not allowed to be there, and be ready to report a crime called "harboring a minor." Otherwise, your kid can stay there and cool off, but once home, the child is back on schedule. The child doesn't get to come home and plop in front of the TV. And the child hasn't earned any exceptional weekend activities. If you are afraid your runaway is suicidal or may hurt someone, call 911. Don't mince words. Tell the 911 operator your child has run away and is *suicidal*; otherwise, the police will have more serious things to worry about.

The most effective way for parents to teach their children is by example. By not accepting disrespect from their children, parents are showing that the kids, too, should have the expectation of being respected by others. By not putting up with violence and by not being manipulated by someone who is threatening to hurt them or threatening self-injury, parents are teaching that children should set the same limits in their own lives. And by putting children in the hospital who need to be there for their own good, parents are showing children that it is okay to need—and get—help.

12

Presenting the Schedule to Your Child

If you believe that people have free will and if you believe that forcing someone to "behave" is not actually the same thing as good behavior (two ideas that I have stressed in this book), then the phrases "He has to study" or "She has to clean up her room" must be qualified. A child has to *only if he or she wants to pass inspection*. And that is a decision that is not under your control as a parent. Language is powerful. If children hear "you *have* to," they may shut you out before you finish explaining what you mean.

When it comes time to present the schedule—which, after all, represents a new way of interacting with your child—try talking instead in terms of what you *want* the child to do. Instead of immediately threatening to take rewards away, explain the concept in language such as "If you want this reward, this is how you earn it . . . but it is up to you." Try not to end statements with the one-word question "Okay?"— for example, "We're going to start the schedule tomorrow. Okay?" You don't want to give your kid the option of saying, "No, frankly, it's not okay."

When I introduce this system to kids, it takes about five minutes.

DOCTOR: Do you like having your parents on your
back?

MICHELLE: No.

DOCTOR: And do you think your parents enjoy being
on your back? [Sometimes kids actually seem to believe parents do. It is up to parents to let their child
know that they hate it.]

DOCTOR: So, if everybody hates it, why does it happen? I can tell you why it happens. There are
two kinds of things in life, things that are fun and
things that aren't. Which would a kid rather do?

MICHELLE: Have fun.

DOCTOR: That's right. And if you or anyone else is
doing something fun and Mom or Dad comes
along and says, "Stop having fun and go do something that's not fun," who would want to stop having fun? I'll tell you who: nobody. And that's when
arguments arise. So here is what I have been telling your parents: *Work first and fun later*. It's that
simple. Oh, one more thing, how will your parents
know if you've done the work or not, so they can
say yes or no to the fun stuff?

MICHELLE: They will have to check.

DOCTOR: That's right, they have to check. You do the
job, they check, and you go have fun. That's it. Oh,
one more thing. What if you're in a bad mood and
decide you don't want to do the work? That could
happen. Here is what I have been telling your parents: *Don't tell her to get back in there and do it because
that leads to an argument*. But you tell me, if you
choose not to do the work, should you still get to
do all the fun things?

MICHELLE: No. [Every kid I have ever asked knows
the answer to that question—never mind the

occasional smart remark—because it is just basic justice.]

Then I tell the child: Your parents had a homework assignment of filling in the blanks in a schedule, saying what the work is supposed to be, and when they are going to check, and what the fun stuff is. And if you want to see what they have come up with, you can check it out, see if it looks fair, see if they've given you enough time for everything, see if there is any fun stuff they forgot.

Kids are given an opportunity to get involved in the final draft of the schedule, but only if they want to. They don't have to. The parent can walk a child through the schedule, or the child can read through it. Kids are told they can give input. They can make their wishes known:

- They can ask for a change in expectations: "Can I do this chore instead of that?"
- They can ask for more or less time than you allotted.
- They can ask for a specific reward: "If I pass inspection in the morning, can I have money for a cinnamon roll at snack break?" (A request like that usually gets a yes response, unless the child has been saving up money for things the parents do not want him to have.) "Can I have a friend over every day?" (You can agree or you can suggest a compromise, like once a month. It's totally up to you—and not to your child.)

Kids have no shortage of wants, and they enjoy making their wants known to the person who can grant them. You want to welcome your children's participation in this process because it gives them a sense of ownership, a sense of being part of the process, of being heard. Give them limited choices: Would they like to make bedtime 10:00 or 10:30 on Friday and Saturday? If they say, "How about 11:00?" maybe you say, "Eleven!? Wow! Well, okay, but only for good behavior, of course." You don't have to grant all their requests, certainly not immediately. You can point out that as time goes by, bigger rewards may become possible as responsibility leads to trust and kept promises lead to a good reputation. Can they go to a rave? "Not while you live under our roof."

Not by praise alone but through all the little accomplishments, accompanied by appropriate praise, does a child's sense of mastery grow, as does feeling accepted and self-esteem and confidence. A positive cycle of growth replaces the vicious cycles.

What about children who don't want to hear about any schedule? (Make an extra copy if your child might tear up the first.) Do you insist that children sit down and listen? After all, you have worked hard coming up with a schedule. Let them know that you *want* them to see the schedule. That in itself is an expectation. But can you make them look at it? Can you make them listen?

Here's an opportunity to practice our principles. In wanting to present the schedule, we have captured the larger problem in miniature. The child has been given an expectation: to participate in making the new schedule. If children choose to participate, the payoff is that they may get concessions granted. If they choose not to participate, they lose that privilege. Clearly it is the children's right to know the rules, but what if they stuff their fingers in their ears? In another sense, it is a privilege just to know the rules because if they are broken, ignorance of the law is not going to be an excuse. A state trooper is going to give speeding tickets whether or not people bother to read the posted speed limit signs.

Refusal to participate means the child has lost an opportunity to give input. Go forward with the plan. The schedule is posted; if children want to look at it, they can. What more can you do? There is nothing more to say. Parents have the responsibility and authority to run the house . . . and to make sure that rewards are not stolen. Then, when children ask why they can't have something, you can say, "I'm glad you asked. It's all there on the schedule."

Kids can fail an inspection without even knowing what they were supposed to do, or what the heck an inspection is. But that is only because they refused to find out. Ignorance of the law is no excuse, especially when they positively refused to learn the law. So when you look in your kid's bedroom and say, "That is not a pass," and your child says, "What are you talking about?" you can reply, "I'd be happy to tell you about it at an impromptu family meeting . . . otherwise you can wait for the Friday family meeting and I'll lay it all out for you."

What about the teen who says, "A schedule is total baloney. This idea is from that dumb book you've been reading, isn't it?" And you say: "Yes, it is." Is using a schedule treating your kid like a baby? No, if you want to put a baby somewhere, you pick him up and move him. A schedule is for people who are growing up.

There will be things you ask of your child that are not on the schedule. If it is a recurrent expectation, it should be officially added to the schedule at a family meeting. If your child refuses to honor an impromptu request because it's not on the schedule, let it go. Better to make progress within the boundaries of the schedule than to worry about the situations it doesn't quite capture. You can understand how your child might not feel like doing something extra. You might not feel like doing something extra for him later that evening, either. Still, to forgive is divine.

13

Teaching Virtue

Parents want kids to behave just because it is the right thing. But learning what the right thing is and practicing doing the right thing are processes. A girl I'll call Casey says denying a reward is the same thing as forcing her to do something. That is how she thinks. She doesn't distinguish between the two approaches because they have been used interchangeably. She recognizes neither the reality nor the limits of her freedom. Sometimes she hates herself. Sometimes she thinks she has a right to have or do whatever she wants. Anyone who gets in her way she tries to intimidate or manipulate.

Casey will learn the difference between coercion and earning rewards over time, as the stress level in her house and in her head begins to decrease. That realization won't happen until her frontal lobes are in charge of her limbic system. The only way children can see that they are hurting themselves by not behaving is for parents to be quiet and allow kids to figure it out for themselves. You could shove a hundred-dollar bill toward some kids and say, "Here, take this!" and their first reaction would be "No!" A reward is not a reward if we feel forced to take it.

Coercion leads to a very limited concept of freedom in which freedom means "the freedom to do *what* I want *when* I want!" More particularly, freedom becomes the freedom to say "No" to others when they place demands on us. True freedom, or let us say a greater freedom, is one that develops over time and is disciplined. Only a person who practices diligently will be free to play the piano. A child may demonstrate freedom by refusing to take piano lessons, but by refusing to have limits placed on his freedom in the present moment, the child is setting up future limits; that is, the child will be unable to play the piano. A child who accepts the limits of piano lessons now will have greater freedom in the future. Children who learn to do a good job keeping their room clean, and who do it with a good attitude even when they don't feel like it, will develop habits that will help them in school and will open up more opportunities in the future, such as choice of college or choice of occupation. Children who demonstrate their freedom by dropping out of school obviously are setting limits for themselves. Ironically, people who grow up thinking that freedom means doing the opposite of what they are told become very easy to manipulate by those who would do so. If you want such a person to turn left, just say "Turn right"!

The practice of coercion sets an example for a child, who then becomes coercive with others. Being coercive can make it hard to make and keep good friends. If the child's only friends are also coercive, the child may feel that the only way to keep friends is to give in to peer pressure: I coerce you, you coerce me. We want kids to be able to stick up for themselves. The so-called terrible twos conceal a marvelous fact about human nature. We have free will, and there is a natural push to develop that free will. A two-year-old who says "No" might seem irritating until you realize there will be times we *want* kids to be able to say "No"—for instance, "No" to peer pressure.

It is only after a child has learned to trust that a parent will not coerce him or her that the child will see clearly the consequence of not doing what is expected. The consequence is losing out on something fun. Eventually a child will equate losing a reward with disappointing the parent.

And finally the reward won't matter as much because wanting to not disappoint will become a goal in itself. That is when a child is becoming truly obedient. Finally the child, by now a teenager, begins to be motivated by his or her own vision of the future. The child has become an apprentice.

A slave is motivated by fear. An apprentice, in contrast, obeys the master's direction in order to learn a skill. We need to see kids more as apprentices, less as slaves. But that requires first that they be obedient. Children must have the experience of knowing they will not be forced before they can develop obedience. Kids periodically must hear the loving words "Okay, if that's your choice" and then suffer the consequences. The tough-love philosophy is not about being hard on kids; love is tough because it is hard for parents to let kids make mistakes.

Obedience itself is a habit that is based on trust. Once the habit of obedience has been established, it signifies that a child trusts that the parent is encouraging the child to do the right thing, even if it is something difficult. Then, like an apprentice, the child will learn tasks by doing them.

Having developed the habit of obedience will not cause children to go into the world blindly doing whatever they are told because while they are practicing obedience at home they are developing other good habits. It is for these habits, the virtues, that we want to praise our kids, rewarding them materially but, more important, with positive attention. Here are some of the good natural habits we want our children to develop.

Courage. Reason is in charge of aggression and of fear. In biological terms, the frontal lobes should be in charge of the limbic system. The courageous person is neither passive nor aggressive but confident and assertive. A courageous person knows when to fight, not as a blind reaction, but as a conscious decision to defend what is good. Courage also entails channeling aggressive energy to help us endure, to be patient, even as we hope for relief from struggles. Courage is doing what is right even when it is difficult, like not cheating on a test even if we could. Courage is enduring without whining. We teach children courage by making them wait for what they want and by teaching them that attitude counts.

Moderation or temperance. Reason remains in charge of the desire for pleasure. No one drinks for the express purpose of getting a hangover, which shows how easily our appetites take charge. Moderation means a person partakes of and enjoys the good things of life but knows when to say when. There is nothing wrong with candy or ice cream; it just may not be the right time to enjoy them. The temperate person is not led by emotion. Nor will the temperate person treat another human being as an object for selfish pleasure. We teach moderation to children by making the rewards come at fitting times in fitting quantities and by not letting kids walk all over us.

Justice. It is just to give others their due. Parents are due the respect of their children. Children are *not* due an explanation for every decision a parent makes. Justice deals with rights. If someone has a right to know the truth, we act unjustly when we lie. If we do act unjustly, justice demands that we correct what we can. We teach children justice when we raise them according to the laws of society. It is justice to have appropriate expectations for children. When we inspect their work, we are keeping them honest until they have proved themselves responsible. In inspecting, we are judging, and the outcome of that judgment means either kids earn the promised reward—their due as children—or they don't. Justice requires that we do not let kids get in the habit of stealing what they have not earned.

Prudence. The master virtue is prudence. It is one thing to desire to do the right thing; it is another to know the best choice in a given situation, in real time. "Prudence is the perfected ability to make right decisions." To know what is best, one must have a grasp of reality. Both a bad self-image and a grandiose self-image are distortions. What is needed is a *realistic* view. We need to know, each of us, the truth that we are very precious. As children come to use their frontal lobes more and more, they become more adept at appreciating shades of gray. Children who can stop feeling defensive learn that *there are good things about them but that they are not perfect and that they can make mistakes and still not see themselves as bad.* Prudence is like wisdom: it cannot be taught; it must be learned. We allow children to practice prudence when we provide them with clear choices. Parents who use coercion and feed the addiction to conflict by overreacting are doing things that serve to cloud kids' judgment.

Humility. Being humble doesn't mean putting ourselves down, and good self-esteem is not just thinking highly of ourselves. Once more, what is needed is a *realistic* view of ourselves. People with low self-esteem hide their inner self because they feel weak in a dangerous world. By promoting good behavior, we hope kids will enter a "virtuous cycle." The more challenges kids are able to master, the more confident they feel. As self-esteem grows, the inner self, once hidden in fear, expands, growing closer to the surface, closer to whom the person appears to be on the outside. As kids grow in humility, making mistakes becomes an opportunity to learn rather than to become defensive.

The system I have described in this book is meant to provide a structure for rehabilitating kids who are going down the wrong path. It is not meant to provide an easy answer for every situation. The parent who works this program must also have the prudence to momentarily scrap the program. Listen to your children: There may be extenuating circumstances for why they did what they did. Life is hard for kids as well as for grown-ups. Mercy is compassion shown to an offender. We teach our kids to be compassionate and forgiving by forgiving them.

Conclusion

There is a riddle about a man who was carrying a chicken, a fox, and a bucket of grain. When the man came to a river, he found a boat so small it would hold him and only *one* of the three things he carried. He had to carry each thing across the river one at a time. But how could he do it without leaving the fox to eat the chicken or the chicken to eat the grain?

This book attempts to unravel a similar riddle: how to teach children responsibility without conflict. If you insist that kids meet their responsibilities, you risk conflict. Avoid conflict and you risk allowing your kids to shirk their responsibilities.

The solution is similar to that of the man at the river. He first took over the chicken, leaving the fox with the grain. Then he returned for the fox and carried it across the river. Instead of leaving the fox with the chicken, he took the chicken *back* with him and dropped it off, then carried the grain across and left it with the disappointed fox, and finally returned for the chicken.

In the same way, parents need to prioritize their goals. The initial dilemma was how to improve behavior while avoiding conflict. In dealing with children, we need to avoid certain kinds of conflict because coercion doesn't lead to improved behavior. But other kinds of conflict need to be met head on.

Expectations and Rewards—Again

Prying kids away from pleasurable activities to do work is a lose-lose situation: fighting about the task causes stress, and giving up means that the child is not meeting expectations. When such situations do arise, I hope you will now be less likely to become angry at a child who offers resistance to turning off a video game. Those situations, too, will serve as reminders to the parents to stay organized. This program puts a share of responsibility on the parent as well as the child. Rather than interrupting fun for work, the parent has a schedule in place that puts work before fun.

Kids know how to use expectations as a means of getting rewards. If they want something bad enough, they will ask what they have to do to get it. You want the lawn mowed? The car vacuumed? You got it. And they will earn that reward, fair and square. One thing to notice is that in this case the child is doing the work freely, not through coercion.

The main vicious cycle described earlier in this book resembles a machine that turns on with bad behavior and spits out conflict and stress. We began by considering what is at stake if kids don't get on the right track: stress making illnesses worse; substance abuse; personality disorders. Our goal is to stop the cycle of vice and promote a cycle of virtue.

In many ways, the approach we have been learning is an exercise in improving behavior while at the same time decreasing the amount of correcting we have to do. Being frequently corrected causes kids to feel criticized and reduces the chances they will even hear anyone's advice, no matter how good. Instead, we worked on a plan that looks at expectations and how they are monitored. Instead of focusing first on what to do about bad behavior, we spent time figuring out how to promote good behavior.

One cannot underestimate the importance of promoting

good behavior by having clear expectations. Expectations are not just about chores. Some kids need more exercise. Some need practice calling a friend or relative on the phone or writing thank you letters. Kids don't raise themselves. Love means paying attention to what kids are doing and what they are supposed to be doing. Paying attention is work, but it is a blessed work.

The straightforward, up-front nature of a schedule communicates clearly to kids what they are expected to do and what is at stake. That clarity eliminates the need for them to be told repeatedly what to do and what will happen if they don't. The bottom line of expectations is that if kids won't meet basic expectations, like cleaning up their room, you are fooling yourself if you think they will keep their promises after you buy just one more video game. They will always want more.

The bottom line of inspection is that you have to inspect what you expect.

Correcting Misbehavior: The Linchpin

The middle portion of the big vicious cycle—correction of the misbehavior—is the linchpin in decreasing the number of corrections. All kids misbehave and are corrected for it. We can now point out that the kind of correcting that parents *usually* do is *verbal* in nature. But a behavior rehabilitation program is largely nonverbal. Once the plan is in place, it is known ahead of time that expectations must be met before the fun starts. A schedule eliminates the need to tell kids what to do because they already know.

How else have we decreased verbal correction? When a child fails inspection, a ton of verbal correction is eliminated when parents learn not to insist that the child "get back in there and do it." This idea of not insisting is often misunderstood by parents. I am not saying don't be firm. Sometimes parents need to turn up the volume to let kids know they are serious. There is a judgment call to be made. Are you encouraging, like a good coach, or are you coercing? Kids who routinely resist doing as they are told may be addicted to conflict. For them, anger is a banquet. In that case it would be better to err on the side of not insisting. In that way you will demonstrate your commitment to honoring their freedom, and they will gain a sense of trust.

Expecting a reward system to produce automatic compliance will backfire. Kids don't want to be controlled, even if it means giving up a reward. The man forced to peel potatoes will develop resentment, not a habit. Honoring people's freedom doesn't mean telling them they can either peel potatoes or dice onions but they *have* to do one or the other.

When a reward system backfires, parents get frustrated and kids get a hidden reward of pushing the parents' buttons. The frustrated parent is the one who can't let go. It's perfectly okay to express anger and disappointment as long as your child sees that you are willing to let it go, to allow them to make a bad decision. But, boy oh boy, bad decisions ought to have consequences. The end of many a reward program comes when parents give up and kids sneak the rewards they supposedly didn't care about. Kids will trust and respect adults who honor their freedom, but they must also learn to trust adults to stick to their guns.

Parents need to take a leap of faith that their child will learn to do the right thing. Otherwise the parent is left insisting that the child do right but the child never learns personal responsibility.

If a child passes inspection, that success should be accompanied by praise and a thank you. The concrete rewards will change: Jamba Juice, Starbucks, the mall, the car keys. But positive parental attention will always matter more than anything.

If the child fails inspection, there is no need for a volley of verbal reprimands. Theoretically, there is no need to say much of anything. If the child didn't already know, a shake of your head will serve notice of failure.

To further decrease verbal correction, don't immediately reprimand a child who complains about not getting a reward. Sympathize, distract, or ignore—do whatever keeps things calm. If the child becomes disrespectful or goes for the TV anyway, turn it off. And here you finally open your mouth: "That's one." You could just raise one finger. But now the time for avoiding conflict is just about over: Parents cannot let themselves be bullied. Parents are not modeling passive or aggressive but rather *assertive* behavior.

The day will come when you shout (or say softly but distinctly): "That's two!" and your child will stop and realize you mean business.

Finally, it doesn't matter if an eight-year-old has Tourette's syndrome or a fourteen-year-old has depression; neither one can be permitted to swing a shovel at his family because he is angry. In no case are we, the parents, supposed to start a fight; however, we might need a plan to stop a fight if one breaks out.

Parents tend to confuse short-term goals such as getting a room picked up with the long-term goal, which is to raise a child to become a responsible adult. The overall goal cannot be seen as getting the room clean (if it were, I might recommend avoiding the fight and doing it yourself). Nor can the goal be for parents to *win* by imposing their will on the child. Coercion doesn't help form good habits, but it will breed resentment and demonstrate to the child that bullying pays off. Similarly, the overall goal is not to avoid conflict. Parents don't need to walk on eggshells around their children. The goal is a long-term one: the development of good habits.

Getting Help from a Coach

No parent is expected to be perfect with a system such as the one I am describing. You might need help implementing this program. There will be times when you will not be able to think clearly. A schedule calls for consistency but also for evolution. Parents often can come up with creative solutions for problems that arise. At other times you might need a mentor, a sponsor, a coach of some sort—a counselor or doctor, spiritual adviser, friend or relative who understands these principles.

Your coach should be willing to read this book and to understand the whole program; a little knowledge can be dangerous. A sponsor will keep you honest and remind you of what you have learned when your own emotional state favors overreacting in anger. When you call your coach to complain that you still have to tell your child fifty times to stop doing something, your coach can remind you that you only need to say it three times. And if you're telling your child fifty times to start working, what happened to the deadline? A coach is best available for crises.

Here is an important reminder: It is very easy to believe that you have the schedule in your head. But writing it down is worth the time and effort. The most successful mentor will have a copy of your child's schedule. That way, when you call for help, your mentor can ask where you were in the schedule when all the trouble started. You might realize you weren't following the schedule. That is going to happen. No good kicking yourself. Start fresh, back on the schedule, tomorrow.

How Long Will It Take?

How long will it take to see real improvement? If you count less yelling at your child as improvement, then it can start today. But, mostly, changing old habits takes time. It depends on the child, and it depends on the parent. The more practiced a child or teen is at bad behavior and the less consistent the parent is, the longer it will take. By now, most parents will realize that the descriptions of problems with raising children fit their own lives growing up. Parents who were overly controlled as children will naturally feel a need for control. Parents with low self-esteem will be at risk for needing approval from their children and always wanting their children to see that they are being fair. I love to see a mother in the grocery store who isn't embarrassed when her child collapses in the checkout line because he can't have some candy. Far worse to buy candy for such a child out of embarrassment than to remain calm and not worry what other people think (many of those other people, like me, actually admire the mother's parenting skills!).

There is more than one way to address problematic behavior, of course. If there is a need to follow some of these other paths before or after implementing behavior therapy, improvement may take longer. A child with attention deficit hyperactivity disorder or a mood or anxiety disorder, for example, might need to be treated with medication first and foremost. The first goal for some parents is for their child to develop better insight; these parents seek out a psychotherapist for their child and family. A child who refuses both medicine and talk therapy (and a great number of other expectations) might need behavior therapy before the other therapies can begin. And that requires cooperation between spouses.

Healing the parents' relationship might need to come before behavioral rehab. However, the approach I have described is meant to give parents something to agree on. I hope that by getting parents to cooperate in parenting this book can contribute to the strengthening of their relationships. It may also be that before couples therapy can go forward, parents as individuals may also need help. It takes courage to admit we need help. Insecurity stops children from admitting they need help; the same can be true of parents.

Even if all the pieces are in place, it takes three months to form a habit. When you consider not just your child's habits but your own, you see why my mentor, Dr. Walkup, would tell parents, "If things are 20 or 30 percent better in a year's time, that's a big piece of pie."

Your child is worth every minute.

References

Foreword

Bor, W., and M. R. Sanders. (2004). Correlates of Self-Reported Coercive Parenting of Preschool-Aged Children at High Risk for the Development of Conduct Problems. *Australian and New Zealand Journal of Psychiatry* 38:738–745.

Burke, J. D., D. A. Pardini, and R. Loeber. (2008). Reciprocal Relationships between Parenting Behavior and Disruptive Psychopathology from Childhood through Adolescence. *Journal of Abnormal Child Psychology* 36:679–692.

Patterson, G. R. (1982). *Coercive Family Process*. Eugene, OR: Castalia Publishing.

Sanders, M. R., A. Ralph, K. Sofronoff, P. Gardiner, R. Thompson, S. Dwyer, and K. Bidwell. (2008). Every Family: A Population Approach to Reducing Behavioral and Emotional Problems in Children Making the Transition to School. *Journal of Primary Prevention* 29:197–222.

Scaramella, L. V., and L. D. Leve. (2004). Clarifying Parent-Child Reciprocities during Early Childhood: The Early Childhood Coercion Model. *Clinical Child and Family Psychology Review* 7:89–107.

Introduction

p. 2 "The science behind this book is based largely on the research of Gerald Patterson." Patterson, G. R. (1971). *Families: Applications of Social Learning Theory to Family Life*. Champaign, IL: Research Press.

p. 2 "The *Journal of the American Academy of Child and Adolescent Psychiatry* calls these evidenced-based principles among the most substantiated in the field." Practice Parameter. (2007). *Journal of the American Academy of Child and Adolescent Psychiatry* 46:136.

p. 2 Thomas, C. (2006). Evidenced-Based Practice for Conduct Disorder Symptoms. *Journal of the American Academy of Child and Adolescent*

Psychiatry 45:109–114. (Thomas cites Patterson as the source of most evidence-based techniques.)

Chapter 1. When Is a Problem a Problem?

p. 15 "... some people are ... simply not good at learning from mistakes." Klein, Tilmann A., et al. (2007). Genetically Determined Differences in Learning from Errors. *Science* 318:1642–1645.

p. 19 "Kids with a bad reputation feel they are unaccepted, which leads to depression." Evans, D., et al., eds. (2005). *Treating and Preventing Adolescent Mental Health Disorders*. New York: Oxford University Press, 16.

Chapter 2. Illness, Stress, and Personality Development

p. 25 "Many kids with learning problems such as attention deficit hyperactivity disorder (ADHD), for example, develop more behavioral problems than can be explained simply by the learning disorder alone." Bombauer, K. Z., and D. Connor. (2005). Characteristics of Aggression in Clinically Referred Children. *CNS Spectrums* 10:709–718.

p. 26 "... stress also affects biology. Headaches, high blood pressure, weight gain, asthma, skin conditions." Stress Symptoms: Effects on Your Body, Feelings and Behavior. http://www.mayoclinic.com/health/stress-symptoms/SR00008_D.

p. 26 Kleyn, C. E., et al. (2007). The Effects of Acute Social Stress on Epidermal Langerhans' Cell Frequency and Expression of Cutaneous Neuropeptides. *Journal of Investigative Dermatology* 128:1273–1279.

p. 26 Bloomberg, G. R. (2005). The Relationship of Psychologic Stress with Childhood Asthma. *Immunology and Allergy Clinics of North America* 25:83–105.

p. 26 "A clear connection exists between stress and depression in children and adolescents." Evans, D., et al., eds. (2005). *Treating and Preventing Adolescent Mental Health Disorders*. New York: Oxford University Press, 12–14.

p. 27 "... stress can cause certain genes to express themselves that would not otherwise be expressed." Minde, K. (2002). Effect of Disordered Parenting. *Child and Adolescent Psychiatry*, ed. Melvin Lewis. Philadelphia: Lippincott Williams and Wilkins, 479–480.

p. 27 Ogren, M. P., and P. J. Lombroso. (2008). Epigenetics: Behavioral Influences on Gene Functions, pts. 1 and 2. *Journal of the American Academy of Child and Adolescent Psychiatry* 47:240–248 and 374–378.

p. 28 ". . . antisocial personality disorder . . . borderline personality disorder." Helgeland, M., et al. (2005). Continuities between Emotional and Disruptive Behavior Disorders in Adolescents and Personality Disorders in Adulthood. *American Journal of Psychiatry* 162:1941–1947.

p. 28 ". . . self-injurious behaviors like cutting themselves." Briere, J. (2001). Self-Injury and Mutilation. Paper presented at the Twentieth Annual Conference on Child Abuse and Neglect, April 10, Sacramento.

Chapter 3. A Parent's Dilemma

p. 38 "Gerald Patterson . . . wrote a field-defining paper showing how a lack of parental monitoring is the final common pathway to juvenile delinquency." Patterson, G. R., et al. (1989). A Developmental Perspective on Antisocial Behavior. *American Psychologist* 44:329–335.

Chapter 7. Putting Together a Schedule

p. 65 ". . . emotional intelligence." Goleman, D. (1995). *Emotional Intelligence*. New York: Bantam.

p. 84 "State-of-the-art residential treatment provides behavior modification much as we have been describing, but in a locked setting." Bleiberg, E. (2004). *Treating Personality Disorders in Children and Adolescents*. New York: Guilford Press.

Chapter 11. Troubleshooting

p. 120 "I teach kids four techniques to use when being bullied." Burnett, K. (1999). *Simon's Hook: A Story about Teases and Put-Downs*. GR Publishing.

Chapter 13. Teaching Virtue

p. 144 "Prudence is the perfected ability to make right decisions." Quoted from Pieper, J. (1975). *The Four Cardinal Virtues*. Notre Dame: University of Notre Dame Press.

Index